CW01460486

Crotch

Height

Perspective

By Steph Derham

Crotch Height Perspective
Contents

Please allow me to introducing myself

Please allow me to introduce myself. My name is Steph. I was born with the condition known as Spina Bifida and I am writing to tell the world about my life as a disabled person living in a non disabled world. This is by no means intended to be a book of self pity or of being a victim. It's a story of changing times and acceptance, in the medical world, the law and in people's minds. My book is intended to be honest, humorous and at times bittersweet. The title is "Crotch Height Perspective" as I believe this suggests to you an insight into how it is to see everything around you at Crotch Height. I hope to make you smile, frown and maybe shed a small tear but above all I hope to show you that we are all still people on the inside, no matter what you see on the outside.

My story begins in 1961 when my mum gave birth to me and my parents were given little hope that, even if I were to survive, I would ever even sit up.

My story hasn't ended. I'm still here. Why am I writing this now you may be wondering Well in 2019, almost 58 years since I was born a mother has introduced to the world the UK's first Spina Bifida baby born following a foetal repair operation to correct the damage caused by this Neural Tube Defect. The operation has already proved successful in other countries but now, finally we have it here.

Statistically 80% of women will abort a baby once told it may have developed Spina Bifida in the womb. I would never pass judgement on these women. This is after all a personal choice. We all have reasons for our actions and that is our business and nobody else's. But what I will say is this. I will be eternally grateful that my own mother wasn't given that choice. Thanks for having me, mum x

How I began

1955-1961

I'd like to tell you how I began. My parents met in 1955. Bob was a 23 year old Articles Clerk and training to become a Chartered Accountant. 17 year old Jennifer was a typist. They met when Jennifer was meant to be on a blind date with Bob's friend Keith. Bob and Keith went to Wyggeston Grammar School for Boys, as did Sir David Attenborough. This was a fact that my dad loved to boast as a sort of mini claim to fame. Keith was training to be a Chartered Surveyor. To Jennifer these seemed very glamorous professions as her humble background was very different. In fact, Jennifer was expelled from her secondary school, just off Fosse Road South in Braunstone, Leicester at the age of 15 for refusing to remove a headscarf when instructed by the headmistress to do so. She had been raised by her paternal grandparents from the age of one as her own mother was accused of neglecting her. This is a fact she was unaware of until she needed a copy of her birth certificate prior to starting work. When she discovered that her "brother" was her father, and her "parents" were her grandparents!

Bob's first words to Jennifer were "Would you like to see my cigarette trick?" And that was it. Jennifer was smitten for ever after. The trick was to hold a cigarette between the middle and forefinger of his left hand and sweep his right hand over the top making the cigarette disappear. A trick that impressed Jennifer at least!

The courtship was hard for both as Bob was working towards gaining his qualification as a Chartered Accountant and this entailed being away from Jennifer and Leicester for weeks at a time, staying in various hotels and B&B's up and down the country. They wrote to each other constantly and Jennifer stored her loving letters from Bob in a sweetie tin in her bedroom. Whenever he was home, they courted at the Roxy Cinema just off Narborough Road on Fullhurst Avenue. They would sit in the back row, holding hands and watching films such as Carousel with Gordon Macrae and Shirley Jones or High Society with Jennifer's idol, Frank Sinatra.

They married on 19th July 1958 and spent a week honeymooning in Bournemouth. Married life began at Bob's mother's house in Bodnant Avenue, Evington in Leicester. Hilda was a widow as Bob's father, a WW1 veteran, had died when Bob was just seven years old from Lung cancer. Bob's sister was at University in Norwich training to be a teacher and his brother was also training to become a Chartered Accountant and was married to Olga. And so it was just the three of them, Hilda, Bob and Jennifer until 24th April 1959 when exactly nine months from their wedding day Jennifer went into labour with their first child. Jennifer's ideal was to be married and have two children, first a boy then a girl. They didn't have a car and so the journey to Bond Street Nursing home was by way of bus. Bob, a smoker, persuaded her to climb to the top deck so that he could have a cigarette on the way. As a non smoker at the time I can only imagine her annoyance. In fact it's a story she was to repeat many times over the years often told with humour when she wanted to get her own back at him for any reason.

Bond Street Maternity Hospital had been converted from six terraced houses sometime in the 1930's. The living rooms were converted to become tiny two-bedded wards where the babies shared the rooms with their new mothers. It had its own milk bank with milk donated by local mothers. Mothers stayed for ten to 14 days, the first five of those confined to bed after giving birth. Jennifer did not stay for ten days. Christopher James (Chris) was small and jaundiced when he was born, and she was encouraged to breastfeed but after a couple of days trying unsuccessfully she developed mastitis and he was reluctantly bottle fed by the nurses. They chastised her and made her feel that she had failed. When Chris was less than a week old she picked up her baby and walked out, discharging herself. She was determined that her next baby would be born at home.

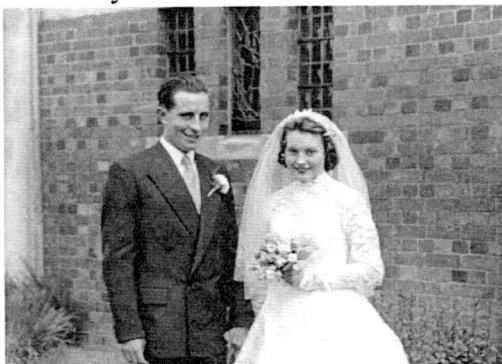

Mum and dad 19th July 1958

Bob and Jennifer had made another step towards the dream, a son. Next on the agenda was to buy their own house. Downing Drive in Evington became their new home. All that remained on Jennifer's agenda was to have a daughter and life would be complete

4

This is me

And so I was born at home on 29th August 1961 in the middle of a late summer heat wave. My mother had a great dislike of hospitals after her experience when Chris was born. Ironic then that after giving birth to me she would spend a huge proportion of my childhood in one, either taking me to appointments or visiting me following the many orthopaedic operations I endured.

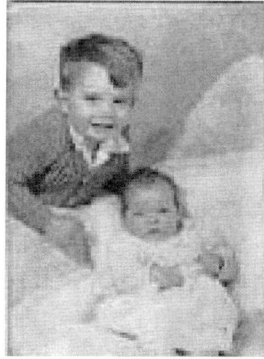

Chris and me

On the day of my birth my brother Chris was taken to the house next door to be cared for by the neighbour, out of the way so that I could make my grand entrance into the world without the distraction of a 2yr old. Dad waited downstairs in the kitchen, busying himself making endless cups of tea and chain smoking. Practising and perfecting his cigarette trick. Once I was safely delivered he was summoned by the midwife and dismissed into the garden with the placenta wrapped up in newspaper so it could be burnt. Meanwhile the midwife spoke to my mother abruptly telling her that she shouldn't worry too much about the bulge on my back. She said that she had seen it once before on a baby she had delivered, a boy, but sadly on that occasion he had only lived for two weeks!! She left and dad went to fetch Chris and came back with ice cream. We were one complete happy family. Obviously mum didn't take much notice of the midwife's words, or if she did she chose to ignore them. She didn't think to question the implications of that lump on her baby daughters back. As you can tell, unlike that boy I did survive. When I was six weeks old I was taken to the local surgery for my check up. Mum told the doctor that she had noticed I didn't really move my legs and wondered why, and when was the swelling on my back going to subside? The doctor said he thought that she understood I had been born with Spina Bifida.

I am Spina Bifida, or I have Spina Bifida, or I was born with Spina Bifida or I got Spina Bifida in the womb!! Which is right? Who knows? To say I am Spina Bifida implies that I own the rights? I have Spina Bifida? To me the whole thing happened months before I was born so surely it should be in the past tense. If people ask I prefer to say I was born with Spina Bifida - it happened and now we can move on and get on with life. I prefer positives. Negatives are so exhausting.

Let me explain as best I can in simple terms. Spina Bifida is a neural tube defect where the spine does not develop properly in the womb causing a gap in the spine. In effect, the neural tube doesn't close all the way. A sac of fluid containing part of the spinal cord and nerves will leak through the opening and they become damaged. This causes varying levels of paralysis along with other complications such as bowel and bladder malfunctions, muscle weakness and loss of sensation in affected areas. There are varying degrees of severity based on where on the spine the defect has occurred. For some babies this could mean brain damage and to others minor impairments. The spectrum is as colossal as the function of the spinal cord.

Since 1991 women are encouraged to take Folic Acid as a preventative measure and are given detailed scans at 20 weeks of pregnancy for early detection. The benefits of taking folic acid were first discovered in the 1920's by scientist Lucy Wills. Following extensive research into anaemia in women she realised that wealthier, middle and upper class women did not suffer from anaemia quite as much and therefore it must be nutrition related. Then in the 1990's scientists discovered that not only did folic acid help with anaemia, it was also beneficial for the development of unborn babies to help prevent neural tube defects such as Spina Bifida. A breakthrough arrived in the UK in 2018 when surgeons successfully removed a foetus detected by scan as Spina Bifida, repaired the defect and returned it to the mother's womb so she may give birth to a healthy baby. This operation had been performed in America and other parts of Europe for several years and finally is now available through our NHS and at the time I am writing this, a total of five operations to far have taken place in England.

An interesting fact is that in the UK 1 in 1000 babies are born with the condition and, as I have said, 80% of all women, who are told at their scans that their baby has Spina Bifida, will terminate. My mum once told me that if she had been told her baby would be born with a disability but that she could terminate, she probably would have done. Now before you all say "How insensitive of her", she followed that by saying, "And what an absolute waste of a life that would have been"

Enough of the biology lesson and back to me!

OK, so no one had bothered to tell my Mum that her baby had been born with a severe disability, so how was she supposed to know? As there was no specialist consultant in Leicestershire in 1961 my parents had to take me on the train to a hospital in Derbyshire. After a full examination and studying my GP's notes the consultant stated that their daughter had been diagnosed as having a congenital birth defect called Spina Bifida. Mum asked the question, "Does this mean then that she won't be able to walk?" to which the reply was "My dear, she will never even sit up". No points for tactfulness there then.

Often Spina Bifida babies are born with open wounds and in those days it was generally considered better to let babies die of starvation rather than attempt to save their lives. I consider three facts probably saved my life.

1. I wasn't born in a hospital.
2. I didn't have an open wound.
3. I was born to a stubborn woman who wasn't going to have any dr or midwife tell her that her daughter was not going to sit up!!!

My Orthopaedic Consultant at Leicester General Hospital was a wonderful man called Mr Tom Stoyle. He often used to quote from a 1944 Academy

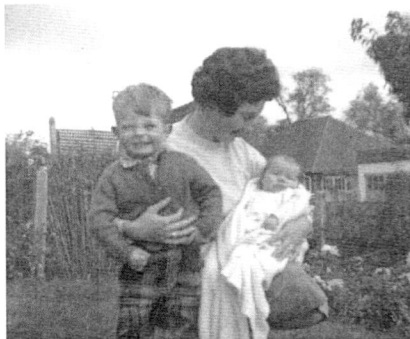

Chris, mum and me 1961

8

Award nominated Song. "Ac-Cnet-Tchu-Ate the positive". For copyright reasons I can't directly quote him (I can't afford the lawsuit!) but the point he was making was a simple one. Concentrate on what is good and ignore what is bad, and don't even consider the bit in the middle!! Between Mr Stoyle and my parents, they made the whole deal a good thing, and I will be forever grateful that Mother Nature decided to give me to my parents and not a couple who would break at the sign of a baby coming from the womb with a lump on her back and immediately think the best option would be a children's home for the infirm (yes I've seen that episode of Call The Midwife). So it happened, we didn't know why so much in those days, but let's deal with it and move on. It's just the way it is!

Hospitals

1961 – 1966

I spent most of the first 5 years of my life in Leicester General Hospital on the children's ward. It was a long nightingale style ward with a variety of cots and beds on each side and a veranda at the end which looked onto the hospital grounds. My parents used to take it in turns to visit. Visiting time was very much restricted on all wards at that time, regardless of whether you were a small child or an adult. Nowadays parents can stay with their child, sleeping on camp beds if they wish. Not so then. My first memory of that time was when a nurse smacked me. She said I wasn't being helpful whilst she was trying to make my bed. When mum came to visit I was crying. Well that nurse must have wished she had taken the day off that day. My formidable mother said to her "How big are you??? And how small is she?? How the hell was she stopping you from making her bed??" Another time a nurse promised me sweets if I promised not to cry when my mum left me after visiting time. I didn't cry and she gave me the sweets. I ate them, and then cried!

I can still remember the smell of those corridors in that hospital and mum or dad carrying me past the operating theatres to get to the children's ward on the day of each admission. The pre med was a pink medicine. Oh how I hated that stuff. On waking from the anaesthetic mum would always be there with a box of After Eight Mints and a bottle of Lucozade. The nurses would give me a drink of tea from a baby beaker. Whenever I have tea now from a plastic cup it reminds me of that post op drink.

When I was born both of my hips were dislocated. I didn't know this until years later but I can remember spending months in a "frog" plaster. My legs were angled so that the hip joint could be forced into the sockets and held with plaster of Paris that went from my ankles to my tummy. My knees were bent and positioned at an angle that resembled frog's legs. And that explains its nickname. A bar was placed across the middle and a hole cut out so that I could have my nappy changed. I have no idea whether the hip situation was related to Spina Bifida but I'm guessing it must be all part of the same development issues that occurred in the womb. Apparently I still have dislocation on my left hip so it wasn't really a complete success.

Another one of my early operations involved removing muscle from my thigh and transplanting it into my lower legs and feet. My feet dropped straight down and the transplant meant that they would be pulled up to sit at 45 degrees to my leg. After the transplant metal plates were inserted to keep the muscles in place until they were fully established and the operation deemed successful. Unfortunately someone forgot to take them out again and in my early 20's I kept getting infections in my right leg. It would start with flu like symptoms, and then a lump would appear in my groin. This would be followed by redness and swelling in the leg. I was attending my cousin's wedding in Norwich once when this happened and my Uncle took me to Norwich Hospital. They x-rayed me and asked about the plates. I was five when they were inserted so really didn't really know much about them or what they were for. Mum explained to me why they had been put there but she wasn't sure why they hadn't ever been removed. A course of antibiotics sorted it though and I forgot about them again.

Another recollection of those early hospital years was from 1966 when I was nearly 5 years old. It was dad's turn to visit but there was a slightly important football match on that night between England and Germany. Mum visited instead and never let me forget (jokingly of course) that my dad wouldn't visit me the night England won the World Cup.

Early memories of family life

1964-1967

My earliest memory of all is me sitting on the floor near a bay window and I had my leg in a full length plaster of Paris. My toes were exposed though and I can remember a big black cat licking my toes!! I must have only been about three perhaps. Although I saw a programme recently about babies development and apparently the reason we have no memory of being a baby is because the part of the brain necessary for early memory doesn't develop until a child is four years old. I guess this is why we can't remember the trauma of being born.

By the time I was aged between three and four before starting school anyone I encountered outside of the home believed I was mute. This frustrated the hell out of mum. It wasn't until adulthood when watching *This Morning* that I discovered this was an actual recognised condition.

"Selective Mutism" is a complex childhood anxiety disorder characterized by a child's inability to speak and communicate effectively in select social settings, such as school. These children are able to speak and communicate in settings where they are comfortable, secure, and relaxed."

So that was me. I just couldn't get any words out. It was impossible. The only people that heard me speak were mum and my brother, Chris. Even my dad had to stand outside the door if he wanted to hear me. I didn't want to be like that, I just couldn't help it. I think I was afraid people would laugh at me. I used to have physio at the hospital and I never uttered a single word every time we went. In shops, whenever people spoke to me, I wanted to answer but words would never come out. Mum would get so impatient and cross with me. When she asked me why? I just said "I don't talk in places" Nowadays I probably would have been referred to a child psychiatrist but back then it was just thought to be weird. I'm pretty sure she thought I was doing it on purpose. I vividly remember the day it all went away. Mum used to go to the hairdresser once a week and Chris and I would go with her. The hairdressers thought I couldn't speak too. Chris went to the shop next door to fetch some sweets for us. He bought me a sugar mouse. I must have forgotten everything else for a moment and squealed in delight "A Mouse"! Everyone in the salon laughed and mum gave me a huge cuddle.

And that was that, nothing bad happened to me because I had spoken in public and from that moment on I've never stopped talking. Some may say that sugar mouse has a lot to answer for. If I were to analyse it now, knowing the stuff that we do about anxiety problems, it may have stemmed from separation issues from spending so much time in hospital away from my family. We may never know.

In 1967 when I was about six years old we moved house. This would be our third home. The previous home was a bungalow but this house was a two story four bedroom one and my bedroom was on the first floor at the front. Dad would carry me up the stairs if he was at home. If not I could scramble up them but then coming down would be achieved by using my hands to crawl on my tummy head first, and quite quickly too. Scared the hell out of people visiting but mum and Chris knew I had it all under control. You see it was all about the independence. I didn't want to wait to be carried. If I wanted to play in my bedroom then I needed to be able to get to it when I wanted and not have to ask for help. Chris didn't have to ask anyone so why should I. I had a record player in my bedroom where I would sit and play Sandy Shaw, The Beatles and listen to the musicals

Oklahoma, Carousel and My Fair Lady. I would imagine that I was an actress / singer / dancer and in my head I was on stage in front of my adoring fans with not a crutch, calliper or wheelchair in sight. I remember my wallpaper being dark blue with pink ballerinas. When they were selling the house I would sit outside the room and refuse to let viewers in until my parents agreed that when we moved they would put the same wall paper up in the new house. They never did! Then we got our first colour television and really moved upmarket and I was worried that if we watched it too much the colour would run out.

During the time in this house a local paper called the Leicester Chronicle did a feature write up on us. I don't know why. But I remember the headline *"A wheelchair at the door but a happy family in the house"* Looking back and thinking about this you have to ask the obvious question. Why wouldn't the family be happy? Does having a disabled child automatically thrust you into a life of hopelessness and despair? Well maybe in some families, but it certainly wasn't the case in mine. From what I can remember of the article it started with the line "Petite and pretty Mrs Jennifer Pollock greets me at the door with a warm smile" What was the reporter expecting?? A sobbing traumatised wreck wearing a black veil and wailing woe is me?? The reporter had asked me what I wanted to be when I grew up and I said a nurse. The actual article said that although I said I wanted to be a nurse, the reporter felt that this was probably because I wanted to be able to pay them back for all they had done for me! Or maybe I just said whatever the first thing was that came into my head. In Fact I didn't want to be a nurse. I wanted to be a teacher.

My parents enjoyed a good social life. We had a babysitter called Gaynor who was lovely. I remember her being so pretty with long wavy auburn hair and freckles. When she got married she asked me to be one of her bridesmaids. As I couldn't carry a posy very well the florist made it into a round ball with a ribbon attached that I wore round my neck.

After Gaynor, the son of one of my parent's friends had the job of babysitting me. One night when he was carrying me up the stairs he touched me inappropriately. I was seven years old but I knew it was wrong. After that I never let him carry me. I clambered up the stairs myself and never did mention it to anyone. Well until now, of course.

Chris kept pigeons and one morning he got up to find a cat had got into the coup and all his pigeons were dead. That's only one of two occasions when I remember seeing him cry. Crying was a weakness and we must be strong. No crying allowed in our house unless exceptional circumstances. Mum was quite clear on the "No crying policy". I guess losing all your pets in one night could be considered exceptional. The second time I saw him cry was when Mum died. Chris and I were only two years and four months apart and yet we only ever spent about one year in the same school. He started at Glenfield County Primary School but the teachers told my parents they thought he was "backwards" Parents weren't having any of that so they took him out of there and paid privately for him to go to Stoneygate School for Boys on London Road in Leicester. I don't think he was "backwards" I think he just didn't like School.

Things my brother taught me:

Never eat the gristle bits from around a fried egg - you will die

Never travel on a blue bus - It will crash

Never stop on a yellow box junction in the road - you will get measles

I remember him trying to get me to walk. He said I should try and walk a few steps then he would go and fetch mum and dad and they would be so pleased they would probably give me sixpence. Cute! One day, Chris and his mate decided they would take me carol singing. We set off with me in my wheelchair and they pushed me from door to door. At each house we sang and then when the door was opened Chris would tell them. "We are collecting for the local Spina Bifida" This would have worked but they wouldn't share it with me so I snitched to mum. No one was using me unless I was going to benefit.

To justify this to mum when she confronted him he said, "Well we were but just cutting out the middle man" She made him give his ill-gotten earnings to the local Spina Bifida Charity.

First Schools

1966-1970

In 1966 shortly after my fifth birthday I started Glenfield Primary School, I didn't qualify for an NHS wheelchair as they considered me too young to need one. They were an expensive commodity. We didn't have the finances to buy one. If I had my choice I would have crawled everywhere. Frankly I'm lucky to have been allowed to attend school at all. My local primary school would only accept me as a pupil on the understanding that I didn't stay for dinner. I'm not sure why this was, but presumably the teachers didn't want to have to carry me to and fro. Mum faced two choices. Home school me or accept the schools condition. Home schooling wasn't really an option for mum; it would mean I was having special treatment.

As with many things associated with that time, the phrase "It's just how it was" comes to mind.

My mother would come and pick me up, carry me to the car and take me home. Then return me back to school again an hour later. She never seemed to mind though. At least it was a "normal" life to be able to go to a "normal" school with "normal" children.

However, there is one very important day around this time. The day mum was carrying me through the school car park, she tripped on a pothole and once again was faced with two choices.

1.   Drop me and save herself
2.   Hang on to me and take the fall

Next thing you know, we're back inside the school, mum covered in blood and being lectured on why she shouldn't be carrying me. Note, by the same people who had insisted I be taken home for dinner knowing I didn't have any other option than to be carried and the only reason I was being carried through the car park at lunchtime in the first place was because they wouldn't let me stay. Through a combination of school policy and NHS procedure I'm not sure what else she was expected to do. It was that day that discussions began. Discussions that were to bring me my first wheels and my road to real independence began.

My dad was working as Company Secretary for Corah, which was a large hosiery manufacturer in Leicester, and they bought me my first wheelchair so that mum would no longer have to carry me.

After my first year at Glenfield Primary School when we moved house this entailed a change of school to Glenfield County Hall Primary School. The house was two doors from the school and I suspect the reason for the move was to make getting me to school easier. It wouldn't involve lifting a wheelchair in and out of the car for my 5ft petit mother. So at seven years old I could walk to school with my big metal callipers, surgical boots and crutches. If I fell over mum would say "come on get up". She would stand, arms folded, and wait till I picked myself up. Other mums and children would watch with shocked faces but she knew what she was doing. All part of the programme to make me independent for which I was, and I still am, massively thankful for.

School milk in those little bottles with silver foil tops. Oh how I hated that stuff. It was always lukewarm and disgusting. I had a friend called Jennifer who lived a few streets away. I used to tell Jennifer to drink mine which she dutifully did. Jennifer used to wait on me hand and foot. I wasn't very quick at getting around so she would walk slowly at my pace, very patiently. I wonder if she became a nurse when she grew up? The headmistress placed a chair outside of her office with a note "This chair is for Stephanie Pollock only" It was for me if I got tired walking along the corridor at any time. And I was very grateful for it. Clunking about with all that metal from the callipers and crutches is pretty exhausting for a seven year old. Could this have been a forerunner for "Reasonable Adjustment" perhaps?

Next door to our house on the left lived a family with three boys and to the right a family with three girls. Sadly I don't remember their names but I was friends with the middle girl who was in the same class as me. When I was eight we had sports day at school. I thought I couldn't take part but my friend insisted. We worked out that the only activity I could take part in would be the wheelbarrow race. She partnered me and held my legs whilst I ran on my hands as fast as I could. We won of course because I was used to the crawling method I'd developed previously. Although the little winners shield was to be shared, she let me keep it. Maybe she also became a nurse.

Getting about

I had my first pair of crutches, at six years old, and they were like a tripod and not the one piece stick that you see today. They didn't go to my elbow but just had handles. A friend of Dad's thought they looked good fun, until he used them as a gymnastics aid and broke his arm. A constant irritation throughout my life has been people wanting to play with my crutches or wheelchair! People, please be aware, they are NOT toys! Would you play with someone's legs without being asked? The next crutches I remember didn't have just a single stick either, but at the bottom a rocker - quite a sensible idea really, except that the rocker would come loose and drop of. This was usually at the most inopportune moment such as nowhere near a seat.

In the house and garden at home I didn't use the crutches. I got around by crawling everywhere. And boy was I a fast crawler. I had my own method which fascinated some. I didn't place my palm flat on the floor. Instead I'd rotate my wrist outwards so that my thumb and bent forefinger took the brunt. I could then drag my legs behind me. I did this right up until I reached my teens when I decided I wanted to be upright. Crawling was just not ladylike. Plus it played havoc with my clothes but to me it was just a quick and easy way to get about so it made sense.

When I was seven or eight Mr Stoyle (Orthopaedic Consultant at Leicester General Hospital) said I should have callipers and special shoes. Like Forrest Gump but they went all the way up my legs to the top. They had numerous straps and buckles and metal bits that clipped inside the special leather boots. They had hinges at the knee to enable them to bend when sitting. I couldn't do it though. They were too stiff. They were heavy, ugly and I hated them. It was dad's job to get me in and out of them. I clunked around in them with my crutches but I couldn't wait for dad to take them off. Then I could get back to crawling and be happy again.

After a couple of years Mr Stoyle changed his mind and let me wear knee high callipers. They were also metal and leather and fitted into the special boots and I could put them on myself. One of my favourite things to do was to take mum's pretty shoes or sandals or even high heels and put them on my hands. I would go into the kitchen where it was a tiled floor and pretend I was walking around, the shoes on my hands making lovely clip clop sounds as I crawled around. I would imagine being grown up, crossing my arms as if crossing my legs etc. It's the closest I've ever got to wearing high heels. I could drift into my imaginary world, dreaming of the sling backs, heels, platforms and open toed sandals I would never get to wear. The boots, or surgical boots as they called them, were made to measure out of the softest leather and probably cost an absolute fortune to make. I could have any colour I wanted so every time I chose a different colour. One day my Dad took me shopping and bought me a pair of black patent little girls' shoes. Highly impractical and I could only sit still with them, not walk about, but I loved them. I didn't crawl for fear of scuffing them but was happy just to own a proper pair of shoes. Once they tried to make the surgical boots look like trainers by putting strips of a different colour on the sides. They looked stupid if I'm honest but nice thought.

I developed my own walk too. Instead of using the crutches how they were intended, ie the way they teach you to use them one foot at a time; I found it quicker and easier to swing both legs at the same time. I forgot where I was one day and I swung into my Mr Stoyle appointment. He was not happy and he shouted "WALK NOT SWING" The clinic was not held in a hospital consulting room as they are now, it was held in the middle of the Children's ward. He made me "Walk" up and down the ward as punishment. I never forgot again and in fact Mr Stoyle appointments were the only times in all my crutch using years that I ever did it his way.

Some years later I was given my first "cosmetic callipers". These were moulded by plaster of Paris from my own legs and feet and then made using a sort of white plastic with Velcro straps. They were designed to fit inside the surgical boots. This meant losing the metal and leather ones, for more subtle callipers, hence their name "Cosmetic". The problem with them was that when my legs get too warm they swell. In hot weather particularly, plastic packed tightly against skin is not a good combination and I would often get pressure sores that would ulcerate. I don't have good circulation and virtually no feeling below the knee so I wouldn't necessarily know there was a problem until it was too late. The problem with poor circulation is that it's difficult to heal.

Wheels

Because I couldn't ride a bike like my brother, mum and dad bought him a tricycle so that he could "croggy" me. In other words I could sit on the front and he would pedal me up and down the front garden. Then dad knew a man called John whose son was also born with Spina Bifida. John had designed and made for

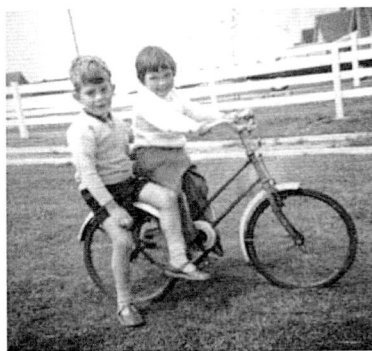
Our trike

his son a hand operated Go-Kart. He made me one too. It was operated not by foot pedals, but by a push pull handle that I operated with my hand. I don't know if the man patented it but he should have. The Hand Controls that they fit on cars to enable disabled people to drive are based on the same design today. I loved it. It was my very own "bike" and my first step to mobile independence.

In 1966 I got my first wheelchair. It was an Everest and Jennings. An E & J was the creme de la creme of wheelchairs and very expensive. A very heavy and cumbersome chair but miles better than having to be carried everywhere. It was bought for me by my dad's employers, Corah in Leicester following my mum's fall carrying me in the playground at Glenfield Primary School. And then in 1968 I qualified for an NHS wheelchair. I was seven years old and too big to be carried anymore, plus I had outgrown the Everest and Jennings one. It was a bright blue affair.

By the time I got to secondary school in 1972 I had learnt how to use the wheelchair as an accessory not a necessity.

The idea was to minimise as much as possible. Remove all side arms, foot plates and make the brakes entirely useless. The chair was just an inconvenience so needed to be as minimalistic as possible.

Over the years I have been asked too many times, "Why don't you get an electric one" to which my response has always been "because it's my legs that don't work, not my arms" Only someone who doesn't understand wheelchairs would ever ask that question. Electric wheelchairs weigh a ton and are bulky. Electric wheelchairs cannot be placed in the boot of a car, or have parts removed to make storage easier.

At nine years old dad took me to see a man in Northampton who was trying to develop a different type of wheelchair. The nice man gave me a prototype and asked me to try it out. The seat was blue and white striped canvas and it looked like a small deck chair on wheels. We (my family) all went on holiday to Spain and I used the prototype for a fortnight. It failed. Some sort of problem with the wheels that kept buckling. Dad took me back to the nice man in Northampton and explained the problem. That nice man was Owen Maclaren. The Maclaren Major Buggy was adjusted accordingly and is still produced I believe, but not a massive success, whereas the Maclaren Baby Buggy is HUGE WORLDWIDE. I like to think I helped Mr Maclaren.

These days, if you can afford it, bespoke chairs are the way to go. NHS Wheelchair Services, a company contracted by the NHS called Blatchford, will provide a voucher towards the cost of a new chair following an assessment. The assessment process will suggest an NHS Chair. In my case NHS is not an option as they can't provide a chair that I would physically be able to lift in and out of my car. (It's all about the independence after all). I had my assessment and Blatchford Wheelchair Services in Leicester gave me a voucher for £850. The amount allocated is very much a "Postcode Lottery" and can vary by hundreds of pounds depending on where in the country you live. I then went to see an old school friend Ian Laker who owns GBL Wheelchairs, and I was measured for a chair that would absolutely suit my needs. Cost a hell of a lot more than £850 but hey, you can't put a price on independence.

On the subject of independence let me tell you about my "bike". Once when on holiday in Tenerife I saw a woman sitting in a wheelchair with some sort of attachment to her chair. I

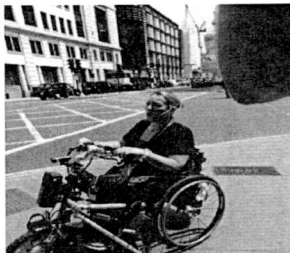
My bike

24

watched her as she wheeled into a restaurant and removed the attachment so that she could stay in her wheelchair and fit comfortably at the table. When she left the restaurant hubby followed her and asked her where she got it from. She said she got it in Germany where she lived. Several years later we did some research and found a company in Milton Keynes that supplied these wheelchair attachments. It is called a Stricker Wheel (named after a guy in Germany who designed it for his own needs). It runs on battery and in effect raises the small front wheels from my chair off the ground and gives my chair an electric wheelchair effect, without the bulkiness, weight and storage problems of an electric chair. Love it. Main thing is that hubby can walk alongside me instead of always being behind. Everywhere I go people stop me to ask about it!!

A man from NHS Wheelchair Services came to service my wheelchair back in the early 1990's and told me he had been repeatedly called to the home of a man who was getting regular punctures. The man later discovered that the reason for this was that his son kept putting darts into his tyres. The son was upset that his dad had to use the wheelchair. You see we don't always realise the impact this can have on our children.

The first time I had a bespoke lightweight chair it was part financed by "Access to Work". A Government funded scheme that assists disabled employees to work. I had to be taught by Rob at Bromakin Wheelchairs in Loughborough (a wheelchair user himself) how to handle it to get it in and out of the car myself. It's a matter of knowing which wheel to unclip first and what position to balance the chair on the car door then the direction to lift. Many times I'm asked by others if they can help and my answer is always the same. "By the time I've explained what you need to do, I may as well do it myself, but thanks"! The reason being, that the wheels and frame have to be positioned on the passenger seat in a certain order so that when I arrive at my destination I can then repeat the process in reverse and get out of the car.

Wheelchair cushions are a head explode too. Who knew there was so much science to it. Depth, density, material, it's not just about the comfort. Hygiene also has to be taken into account. Pressure sores are a common problem for someone sitting down for the majority of the time and this is why all these factors are so important. These pressure sores can become a real problem because how do you take the pressure off in order to allow time to heal. So far I've been lucky but recently I was told by an Occupational Therapist that as I get older my skin will become thinner. So that's something to look forward to.

Often I've been asked the question, "So how long have you been in a wheelchair?"

My reply "Since I got out of bed this morning".

The next move

1970-1971

The problem with all this positivity, independence and normality is that I really didn't understand. As a child, yes I knew that I couldn't get about the same way my parents and my brother and other people around me, but it didn't matter because I could still get about and keep up. The reality only really hit me when I was nine and I changed Schools again. Yes that's right, three primary schools in five years. It was because we had moved house again. To Forest Rise, Kirby Muxloe in Leicestershire

And this time it was very different. Leicestershire County Hall provided me with a taxi to get me to and from School as Kirby Muxloe Primary School was too far for me to walk to or even to be wheeled to. By this time mum had started working for my dad as his Secretary because he had left Corah and set up his own business RL POLLOCK FCA. My parents would leave for work and my brother would catch the bus to his School. Then the taxi would collect me from home, drop me off at school and pick me up at home time, where I would fend for myself until Chris and mum came home. I would make myself sandwiches, apricot jam ones were my favourite and put them on a tray in the kitchen then crawl into the living room pushing the tray along. I would then watch TV – "Nanny and the Professor" with Juliet Mills or the "Ghost and Mrs Muir" were my favourites. Mum would usually be home before dad (yes, we were a two car family) and together we would watch "Peyton Place" with Ryan O'Neal and Mia Farrow together and then she made dinner. So you see, all together a very normal, happy family life.

But at school it was so different. I was put in the class of Mr Derbyshire. He was young and *very pleasing on the eye* according to mum. I would be teased and made fun of. There was a boy in another class who I think had had some kind of road accident and he also wore callipers and walked with a limp. I remember on my first day one of the children seeing me and saying, "Look we've got another one"

There was a particularly nasty group of boys who liked to try and push me over at playtime. The game was to see if they could push me over and then watch me get up again before the teacher saw. Some of the children in my class liked to play with my crutches to my annoyance and one day we had to leave the classroom to go into the hall for something. Everyone left and I couldn't find my crutches. I sat at the table and just waited for them all to come back. Strangely they suddenly reappeared when my classmates returned. Could one of them have hidden them? You may wonder why Mr Derbyshire didn't even notice I was missing. Why indeed.

I never told anyone. I was too embarrassed but it was beginning to become apparent to me that I was different. In PE I would be made to sit on the bench and watch my classmates. Afterwards the children would be sent back to the classroom and I would be allowed to "have a play" on the equipment for a short time. And when I say "equipment" I mean I was allowed to sit on a gym mat and climb over the long wooden beam. Maybe throw a bean bag through a hoop. Stuff like that.

So you see, at home I was very normal and very independent. But at School I was disabled. I didn't tell anyone at home either. It was the "No crying policy" that mum had introduced. No show of weakness. To tell what was happening might have ended in tears. So it was better not to and just get on with it. Keep a stiff upper lip and all that. Doesn't mean I didn't cry, just that I didn't cry in front of anyone. It was exhausting always putting on a front though.

On the 15th February 1971 this country went to decimal currency and I was nearly ten. It was known as Decimal Day in the United Kingdom. I had been in hospital and following an operation had to spend months at home recuperating. The school wouldn't allow me return until I was completely healed. And so consequently I missed all the lessons but Mr Derbyshire sent me some books so I could learn it myself at home. Thank heavens for my parents and my brother who first learnt the changes themselves and then guided me through the process. There was no hospital school in those days, just someone who would come round with a trolley and give you a book or a jigsaw.

One day in 1970/71 a doctor came to our house to make an assessment of me so that my parents could claim a new benefit that had been introduced called Attendance Allowance. It was designed to help people who cared for someone with a disability. Anyway thanks to my upbringing so far, as the independent child who was equal to her brother, they turned me down. Hooray I thought thinking I'd done well to fool him into not seeing that I was disabled. But no, parents, not being happy with the decision, appealed and another doctor came to the house. That morning I'd had a fight with Chris and had hurt my finger. Mum asked this doctor to take a look at it while he was there and he concluded it was probably sprained. He didn't ask how I had come by it and so in his assessment he wrote "She had an injured hand due to a fall" And therefore, this time, parents were granted the Attendance Allowance. I didn't really understand what all that was about, just some doctor asking questions and filling in a form. I was used to doctors and hospitals so it didn't really seem out the ordinary. However, the letter came saying it had been approved. It was left lying on the dining room table. The letter heading read "The Chronically Sick and Disabled Persons Act 1970"

"Why would we get a letter like that Chris?"

"It's for you" Chris replied

"But why"?

"Because you are Chronically Sick and Disabled, you dummy"!

Chris didn't mince his words even at the age of twelve.

So you see, parents had done such a good job of *not* making it a big deal that I still remember the shock and realisation that this was why I was having such a hard time at school. I must be so different from other children. Whilst adults and my family could treat me with normality, it was a difficult task to expect children of nine, ten and eleven to just accept it. Most of them had probably never seen a disabled person before. This was the late 1960's - early 1970's and whilst the children at my previous schools had just accepted me, these kids were fast approaching becoming teenagers. I think looking back that if I had stayed at Glenfield County Hall School, then the children there, who had accepted my differences from the age of six upwards, would have just continued accepting.

In my 2nd year at Kirby Muxloe Primary School I came home with a letter. It was about a school residential trip to a place in Derbyshire. I remember mum speaking to the teacher who was organising it and querying whether I was meant to get the letter. The teacher's said "of course she can come and we will look after her". I loved the trip because it was nice to be away from the school and for it not to be because I was in hospital. I loved the teachers who came with us. But one day we had to go to a graveyard and do some etchings of the gravestones. One little girl called Mandy came up to me and whispered "You're a spastic twit and you belong in that grave" Charming! She was of course reprimanded by a teacher who called her a nasty spiteful little girl. Funnily enough after that Mandy and I became the best of friends.

Time for change

1971-1972

I loved that house in Kirby Muxloe; we had a really long driveway with hazelnut trees either side. Squirrels were constant visitors. Forest Rise was an un-adopted road which meant multiple potholes. Not easy to get up and down in a car let alone a wheelchair or crutches. To the right of the driveway was a small piece of land that no one seemed to own. It was like a bridleway and I have no idea how far it stretched but I do remember playing in it and crawling along it until I got as far as the end of our garden. I think it may have led to a housing estate. Next door to the bridleway was a house that Chris and my friends thought was occupied by a witch. Her name was Mrs Biggs and one day she had an argument with mum where she yelled "Forest Rise was a nice quiet place until you came here, now it's all children and dogs". We only had the one dog but I guess we may have seemed a little boisterous to an old lady. Her house always looked dark and foreboding. I thought it was probably filled with cats and potions. To the left there was a family with boys and their dad was a teacher. I was a bit afraid of him and I don't really think we had much to do with them but next door to him lived a nice family Alison was my age and we played a lot together. One day whilst on holiday her father died of a heart attack. It was very sad and the first time I'd ever encountered dealing with the death of a person.

In the rear garden we backed onto a housing estate and the person who lived in the house nearest to ours was a professional footballer who played for Leicester City called John Schoberg so I was told by dad. Mum had an argument with him because he lit a bonfire and our washing smelt of smoke. On the patio area near the back door I played hopscotch!!! Ok, hopscotch with crutches is tricky but doable as long as your imagination lets you believe you are doing it. Skipping was not, however. It is impossible to hold a skipping rope and crutches but nevertheless, not wishing for me to be left out, my grandma bought me a skipping rope. There was another game that was popular with children then. It involved a length of elastic that you would have two people holding the elastic with their feet and you had to criss-cross a bit like cat's cradle but with your feet. I don't know if children still play stuff like that. I couldn't really do it but I had a go and probably looked a right idiot but only ever did it at home, definitely not in the playground. I was better at conventional cat's cradle that only involved hands.

When I was ten years old my parents decided to take up Badminton. They bought a badminton set and played in the garden. Chris played badminton with them too. They would have tournaments where they took it in turns to play the winner. It was hard. They were doing something that it just wasn't possible for me to be included. It never crossed my mind to use the

32

wheelchair back then to join in. To be honest, I didn't even know where they kept the wheelchair. I felt really hurt. Why would they want to do something that would exclude me? Watching them having fun and knowing that they didn't need me in order to achieve that was so difficult. Looking back now, I see that they didn't do it deliberately but merely to have a hobby themselves. Why should they and Chris miss out just because I couldn't do it? Nevertheless, it was hard and upsetting to me. I felt selfish for feeling like that but just couldn't help it. It was just like the PE lessons at School. Sit and watch then you can play with the racket and shuttlecock when we have finished. Of course I never let on. In my first 10 years of life I had always been included, never felt left out at home. We did things as a whole family and I was no different to any other child. But that badminton set was a real wake up call to how things were going to be in the future for me in life.

Sometimes you just have to accept *"That's just the way it is"* and move on.

My bedroom was upstairs and my Dad would carry me up to bed at night. Outside my bedroom window was a large tree that used to blow in the wind. I was always afraid that one day it would blow down and crash into my bedroom. There was a spare bedroom next to mine that had a large desk in it. I would sit at that desk and pretend I was grown up and at work. I would talk to my pretend colleagues. Mum came up the stairs one day and watched me. She said I looked like I was carrying out interviews!! It was just in my imagination that I was some high flying executive but still very embarrassing to be caught. My parent's bedroom was next to mine the

33

other side and they had big fitted wardrobes where they would hide our Christmas presents. I soon learnt that Christmas day isn't as exciting if you already know what you're getting. Snooping doesn't pay. The bathroom was opposite my bedroom and if I needed to get up in the night I would crawl across and lift myself onto the toilet. One night, I don't know what happened but I fell off and smashed my face on the washbasin. I can only assume I fell asleep but at the time I thought that I had fainted. I shouted for my parents as I lay on the bathroom floor. I couldn't get myself up because I was dizzy and bleeding. They thought the sound was coming from the TV as they were still downstairs so I was ignored for a while. The next day I went to school with a black eye and a cut nose!! Someone said to Mr Derbyshire, "Look at her face" to which his reply was "What's wrong with it, it's a very pretty face" Good answer! I never told anyone what had happened. I just said I'd fallen. That's all anyone needed to know. Falling could happen to anyone but falling asleep on the toilet and not being able to pick myself back up again was different. Falling like that made the disability more apparent and I would have to face up to it, so to me the least fuss the better.

Then in 1972 everything changed for me. Discussions began about where I was to continue my education. At eleven I needed to go to secondary school. Now the options were limited in 1972. Anstey Martin High School was the one for my catchment area and was what they called in those days a Secondary Modern School. My brother was already going there having finished at Stoneygate School. Unfortunately Anstey Martin was built as many secondary schools of that time with flights of stairs between classrooms. At primary school each year group had its own classroom and the

34

teacher came to them, but with secondary it was the pupil that moved to different rooms depending on the subject. Science, Art, Geography etc all in different parts of the school. The practicalities of me getting from one class to the other without missing any of the lessons were unrealistic.

The next option was a school specifically dedicated to children with disabilities.

In Leicester there was such a School that had just opened having been purposefully built in the grounds of Leicester General Hospital. Ideal you would have thought. Except that at that time dad was on the Committee of Leicestershire Association for Spina Bifida and Hydrocephalus and had some knowledge of the expectations for Ashfield School. (Hydrocephalus is a condition that simply put is a build up of fluid on the brain, 90% of babies born Spina Bifida will also have hydrocephalus, I'm in the 10% fortunately) Dad felt that the School was being built to satisfy the legal requirement to educate children until the age of 16, but that the level of education was not going to be of the same standard as other mainstream schools for non disabled children. I have no idea how he came to this conclusion, or indeed whether he was accurate, but he also felt that Ashfield was to be more of an institution than a learning experience. "Somewhere to send her because we have a legal obligation to give her an education" was how dad saw it.

Somehow dad heard of another school which had been specifically designed and built for girls with physical disabilities. This was a grammar school and hence the need to take an entrance exam to qualify to attend. Under the Education Act of 1944 pupils who took an 11 plus exam and passed, could go to grammar school, whereas those that didn't pass went to secondary modern schools. And so I took the exam and miraculously passed, even though I had missed chunks of schooling due to hospital and operations. The next hurdle was to find the funding. Mainstream education is free to children but if you want to opt out then there were school fees to pay. The particular School that dad had his eye on was approx £1000 a year and let's not forget this was 1972. And so he approached Leicestershire County Hall Education Department and asked if they would be willing to make contributions to the fees. Miraculously they agreed to cover all fees. Parents then discussed it with me to see how I felt about leaving my friends to go to a different school. Not really a problem I thought! The real problem was that this School wasn't in Leicester or even Leicestershire. In fact it was 120 miles away in a little village called Holybourne in Hampshire and I would have to leave home and stay there during term time. "Florence Treloar Girls School".

The next stage was to visit the School to see if it would pass father's approval (and mother's of course) Dad had a client who owned a Rolls Royce and the client offered us the use of his Rolls and Chauffeur to take us to Hampshire for the interview. We arrived at Florence Treloars in style that day. We had a meeting with the Headmistress Miss Anderson, who was also disabled. We were then shown around the School by the Deputy Headmistress Miss Barlee. I had never seen so many disabled children in all my eleven years. So many different body shapes and sizes, so many wheelchairs and crutches of different designs. But what impressed me most were the sports facilities. Girls, like me were doing PE (Or Gym as secondary schools preferred to call it) and outside they had tracks painted for racing. And there were canoes hanging up around the swimming pool. I was sold.

And so in the Autumn Term of 1972 at eleven years old my new life began.

First Holiday Memories

1965-1977

My first recollection of a holiday was going to Bullins in Minehead with mum, dad and Chris. I didn't have a wheelchair still so it must have been pre 1966. Dad carried me everywhere. One day he put me on one of those little trains that takes you all around the park and brings you back to where you started. With Chris sitting beside me off we went. Dad was waiting to meet us back where he left us except that when the train returned we weren't on it. You see we had got off at the wrong stop and with no dad waiting my six year old brother then gave me a piggy back while we went to look for him. Fortunately a man who we had seen in the cafeteria with his family at meal times saw us and took over the carrying from Chris, much to his relief. There was a park with a swings and a see saw. Dad sat me on the see saw with Chris and went back to the chalet for something. Chris got bored and wandered over to the swings leaving me still on the see saw but with no one the other side so I was at ground level. Some older girls came along. The girls wanted the see saw and lifted me off, expecting me to stand and walk away. Dad came back just in time to catch me.

We holidayed in hotels in Bournemouth and Ilfracombe. Mum wouldn't fly then so there was no chance of going abroad. Off we would go in the car to our destination. One day we were all on the beach at Ilfracombe and they realised I was missing. I had taken myself off and crawled down to the sea! Well why not? Every summer for two weeks Christopher and I would be taken to Norwich to stay with Aunty Audrey and Uncle Cyril and our cousins Richard and Diana. We would go strawberry picking and to the beach. I can remember Uncle Cyril would carry me onto the beach. Audrey still lives in that same bungalow today and with all the house moves throughout my childhood that bungalow on Reepham Road is the only constant throughout my life. Once delivered Mum and Dad would go off on their own holiday. We also used to congregate in February every year at Reepham Road, when grandma was still alive, for her birthday. All aunts, uncles and cousins would get together and somehow Audrey and Cyril managed to accommodate us all.

At age eight we went to Spain for the first time. Mum still wouldn't fly so we had to drive there. It was a long journey. We would have two nights on a boat and then drive across Spain to the coast. Oh it was hot. There was no air conditioning in cars back then. The first Spanish holiday we stayed in a hotel, Hosteria Del Mar which was in a small fishing village called Peniscola where an Australian guest at the hotel taught me to swim. Mum and I had matching dresses that she made for us. After that we holidayed in various resorts on the Costa del Sol. Sometimes sailing to Spain and other times driving through France. But never flying! Then one day, in 1978 when I was just 17, after watching "Dallas" on TV Mum decided she wanted to go to America. We all know that if we really want something badly enough we have to at least try to make it happen. And so she and dad flew to Miami, leaving me and Chris to fend for ourselves and there was no stopping her after that. I spent most of the three weeks they were away cleaning up after Chris and his mates.

The Treloar Years

1972-1978

If I could say one defining thing that changed my life it was attending Florence Treloar School in Holybourne, Hampshire. I have been asked many, many times if I thought going to a special school and a boarding school at that, was the right thing to do. My reply is always "Yes"

Lord Mayor of London, Sir William Purdie Treloar began a "cripples" Fund in 1907 to help children suffering from Non-pulmonary Tuberculosis (TB). The following year in 1908 he opened a School and a Hospital in Alton, Hampshire so that the children could be moved out of London to cleaner, less polluted air in order to rehabilitate. These were taken over by the NHS in 1948 and the School was moved to the nearby village of Froyle where it became known as Lord Mayor Treloar College for Physically Disabled Young Men.

Florence Treloar was the adopted daughter of William Purdie Treloar. Florence Treloar School was opened in nearby Holybourne on the 24th September 1965 for the education and development of physically disabled girls. The school cost approximately £480,000 to build and could cater for 100 "Able and gifted physically handicapped girls" according to the Trustees. The first girls to attend the school ranged in age from 10 to 18 years and came from 18 different countries. In September 1972 I was the youngest of the 97 girls attending at that time. A week after my 11th birthday my dad drove me, mum and Chris to Holybourne. Mum had spent weeks before this sewing Cash's name tapes "S Pollock" into every item of clothing I owned. As well as my clothes I had a metal tin for a tuck box and a wash bag full of lovely things that she had packed for me including Pears Soap and a pink bubble bath that smelled divine. The rules stated that we had to have our own napkin rings. Mine, of course, was made of silver and was engraved fancily with my initials. But my most prized possession though was my David Cassidy poster.

I had grey pinafores and grey cardigans packed for the winter uniform but the shirts and summer uniform dresses were made by two ladies in the sewing room on the first floor. The colours were olive green, a lilac and a dull yellow.

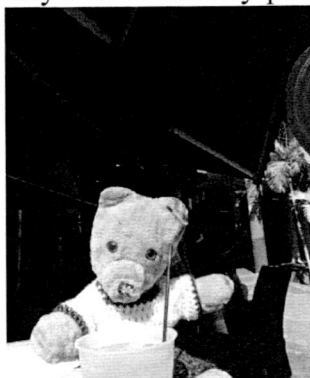

Fred born 25th December 1961

I think it's time that Fred had a mention. Fred is my teddy bear given to me Christmas 1961. When Chris woke up Christmas morning he came into my bedroom and saw Fred sitting astride the side of my cot. "Look, Santa has left the baby

40

a teddy bear" he shouted in delight! Fred has been by my side at every operation and whenever I woke from surgery Fred would be bandaged by the nurses on the same limb that I had been operated on. There was one time that I lost him in hospital. He was rescued moments before entering a boil wash in the hospital laundry, but for the couple of days that he was missing I felt like someone had died. I'd lost my best friend and thought he was gone forever. No, I wasn't a child, I was in my 30's but that's how much Fred means to me. And so of course Fred was by my side as I settled into boarding school life.

We arrived a day late. My parents had misread the letter and when I turned up on the Sunday afternoon we were met by Miss Barlee, the senior mistress, who said "Ah, the missing link has arrived" I was shown to a six bed dormitory on the pink corridor. I was told the pink corridor is for the juniors and the blue corridor for the seniors. The corridor was made up of dormitories of two beds, four beds and six beds. There was a common room and a few bathrooms and right at the end was a self contained flat which the junior house matrons could use.

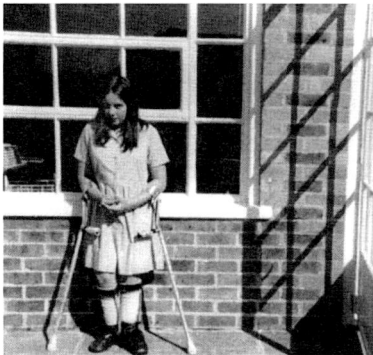
Me, Treloar's girl, such innocence

They helped me unpack. Well mum and dad helped me while Chris stood around looking awkwardly at what was to be my home for the next six years. I wonder what he was really thinking! Would he miss me? Was he happy that at last he was going to get mum and dad to

41

himself without them leaving him with friends and neighbours all the time while they took me to hospital appointments or visited me on alternate evenings when I was being treated? The truth is I don't know, we have never talked about it. Anyway, I was allowed to put my David Cassidy poster on the wall above my bed. The rules were only five items on the dressing table and no sweets or snacks. All tuck tins had to be locked in a cupboard in the Rec room (Recreation room). Every day after lunch we could go into the Rec room where the cupboard would be unlocked and we chose five sweets or one small bar from our tuck tins.

Once unpacked it was time to say goodbye. Quick hug, stiff upper lip and gone! Did anyone cry on the way home after they left me? I don't know, I never asked. All I knew was that I shouldn't cry because that would make it harder for them to leave me. Up until this point I'd only really known Spina Bifida as a disability. I had no idea about any others. After waving my family off I wandered back towards my dormitory and striding alongside me was the smallest person I'd ever seen. I didn't know about the Thalidomide drug that had caused such tragic deformities in babies. I made it my business to find out though and asked mum next time I saw her. I discovered that the drug Thalidomide had been introduced in the UK in 1958 having been developed by a pharmaceutical company in Germany. It was prescribed to pregnant women who were suffering from morning sickness. Use of this drug unbeknown at the time caused limbs to not develop in the baby in the womb and sometimes just a stump in place of an arm or leg. Feet could be upside down or maybe just a couple of fingers coming out of a shoulder, where the arm should be. There were many different deformities' caused by

Thalidomide as it depended on which days in pregnancy it had been taken. The drug was finally withdrawn in the UK in 1961.

Suzanne was about half my height and had no arms, just fingers and upside down feet. But she was beautiful. She smiled up at me, and I will be forever grateful for that smile because straight away I didn't feel quite so lost. I had a friend now. Suzanne had started the day before and was new like me but she had found her way round the school and she looked after me that first day.

I learnt a lot about the different disabilities from my peers during that first term. Some of the girls didn't even appear to have anything wrong with them at all but they had hidden disabilities such as severe asthma, diabetes and epilepsy. Polio was also one of the main causes too. The poliovirus was a major health problem in Victorian times in the UK and continued to be of significant concern for many years following. It was easily spread causing epidemics around the world. Victims could experience spinal and respiratory paralysis. Although incurable, it has been eradicated almost worldwide by a simple vaccine. The vaccine is called "Sabins OPV" and was introduced in the UK in 1962 being given to young children on a sugar cube. This was 1972 and although the Thalidomide drug had been stopped, and we were vaccinating against Polio it was too late for all those children that had been victims. The best that could be done was to provide an education to those children. At the time Florence Treloar School opened in 1965 a fifth of all girls were victims of Polio. By 1975, ten years after the doors first opened three quarters of pupils were wheelchair users, either full time or part time. Of that ten were electric!

It wasn't just the academics they were teaching us at Florence Treloar though. Their aim was to teach us to grow to be independent young women. That first term I became involved in sport for the first time ever. No more sitting watching for me. I could already swim but wheelchair basketball, volleyball and canoeing were all new to me. We were allowed to climb on the apparatus in the Gym and swing from ropes. If we fell, it didn't matter you just get up and carry on. No one was going to make fun or laugh at us. Parents didn't sue schools in those days if their child got hurt. And anyway, parents wouldn't see bruises because by the time they saw us any scars had healed. I joined the girl guides and was made class rep in that first term for the committee that organised the Christmas and Summer Fayres.

One day I noticed my name on the big blackboard outside the Rec room along with 3 other of my classmates. It said to go to the school hall at lunchtime that day.

We did and found that the four of us had been selected to play bridesmaids in the Christmas production of "Trial by Jury" by Gilbert and Sullivan. I couldn't sing but as I'd never been picked for anything like that before I'd give it a go. I didn't realise at the time but obviously I and Amanda were chosen because we had wheelchairs, and Sally and Jenny because they were walkers and it made a neat package on the stage, not because of any talent.

The term was split by one short weekend which ran from Saturday morning after Prep until after tea on a Sunday, a week for half term and then a long weekend which ran from Friday morning until Sunday evening. Leicester was too far away for me to be picked up on a Saturday and returned on a Sunday so that first short weekend parents and brother came to School, picked me up and we stayed at the Post House Hotel in Reading. They had a swimming pool and a lovely restaurant and I enthusiastically told them everything about my first few weeks at Treloars. I told them about Trial by Jury and they laughed. "But you can't sing" "I know but I look the part so it doesn't seem to matter" When they returned me back to school on Sunday evening and drove away, I felt lost again. But by now I had friends and some had not been lucky enough to get to see their families.

A Florence Treloar day would start by the ringing of a hand bell to

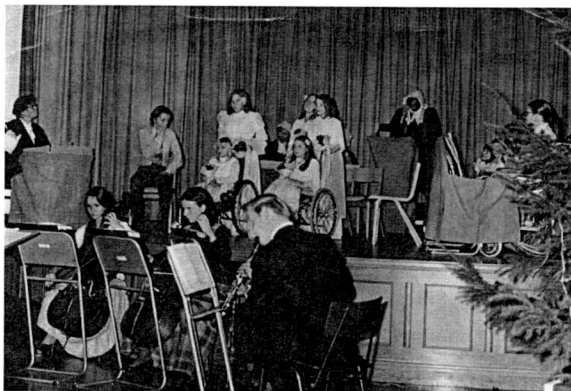

Trial By Jury 1972

wake us up followed by, an hour later, someone shouting "Five to Eight" this meant it was time for breakfast. Each form year had its own classroom so there was less moving about from class to class. The teachers would come to the class, rather than the other way round at "Normal" schools. The exceptions were Science, Music, Home Economics, Needlework, Typewriting and Art that had their own rooms.

45

Some of the teachers were disabled too. The Headmistress walked with crutches and used a wheelchair. I believe she had been a victim of polio

Miss Watson, RE and Needlework teacher wore a metal calliper and limped so I think she may also have been a polio victim. Our history teacher, Mr Matthews wore a hearing aid and rumour had it that Mrs Simpson, English teacher, had no toes. Matron was Miss Hobson and she had been born with a cleft palate.

If you said you had anything at all wrong, headache, upset stomach or a cold it was assumed the main cause was homesickness and Matron would give you a little white pill. A placebo, and send you on your way. If you could actually prove you were ill you were sent to sickbay. Sickbay was like a treat. You could lie in bed all day and watch a small portable TV and have your meals brought to you. Once myself, and a girl called Sandra who was a year older than me found ourselves in sickbay with colds. Once the cold had passed we didn't want to leave so we did everything we could think of to convince matron we were still poorly. We performed fake coughing and sputtering every time we heard her footsteps coming. We pressed up against the radiator to make us hot. We placed bundles of tissues at the side of the bed. The problem was that Miss Hobson had already seen it all before and we were discharged back to our dorms. I remember a girl called Jenny drinking shampoo to get into sick bay and that's the lengths some will go to for a treat!

Going home for Christmas at the end of the first term I was excited. But I had lost touch with any friends I had made at primary school and spent much of the time with family. Mum was impressed with how much more independent I was. Dad no longer needed to carry me up the stairs to bed because I had a new confidence about throwing myself around. I could climb onto the kitchen work surface to make a sandwich or a hot drink. Even though they had tried to bring me up to not think of myself as disabled, it must still have seemed to them that I might never actually be fully self sufficient and so this new found agility may have been reassuring.

PHAB (Physically Handicapped and Able Bodied). When I was in my early teens and in the school holidays from Treloars my parents thought I might like to join a club. At primary school I had been in the Girls Brigade and loved it. I even took part in the "Marching" around the community hall each week. I could keep up with everyone and didn't see any issue at all. Then one of the girls was knocked down by a car and found herself having to use crutches for a while until her injured leg healed. When it was time to march she sat at the side and cried. She sobbed her heart out because she couldn't march. I'm ashamed to say I didn't offer any sympathy. I thought she was just being a wimp and feeling sorry for herself. For goodness sake, what would my mother have said to her! If I can march why is she not even trying was all I thought. I get it now though; it was all new to her whereas it was just so natural to me. Anyway dad dropped me off one night at my first PHAB meeting. This was a group of teens and adults of varying disabilities along with a handful of non-disabled teens and adults. We sat around just talking about stuff and had tea, orange and biscuits. Then dad picked me up and took me home. I never went again. I didn't like it at all and I can't really pinpoint why. It wasn't just that I was in a room full of strangers, feeling like the new girl. It was more that these people weren't from Treloars and to me the only disabled people I wanted to mix with where my school friends.   Away from Treloars I wasn't interested.

I wouldn't say I was academically the brightest in the class. But I coped.   My favourite subject was RE, Religious Education.   Not because I was particularly religious. I just loved the stories.   Second preferred subject was English, both language and literature. But I did not maths, definitely not maths. I was never going to be an Accountant like my dad. We were taught French by a Miss Deavin. She was a petite grey haired lady who looked stern and pushed a trolley loaded with books from classroom to classroom.   She wasn't French but always spoke to the class in French. We were given French names and mine was Therese. Just along the classroom corridor was a small room where Mick the wheelchair man was based. If you had a puncture or a loose brake you had to go to see Mick and he would fix it for you. On Saturday mornings we had to be in the classroom after breakfast for Prep. We didn't have homework obviously so Saturday Prep was the boarding School equivalent. Sunday mornings we donned our straw boaters and walked to the village Church where the Rev Coutts would conduct the service. Spare time would be spent in our common room where we mostly played records and chatted. On a Thursday evening the whole school would try to cram into the Rec room to watch "Top of the Pops". The other purpose of the Rec room was as a waiting room whilst waiting to be called in to Lunch or Evening meal. A sixth former would sit outside the door and wait for the signal from the dining staff.   Once they got the signal they would say "Going in" and we would all pile in.

I made friends for life at Treloars. We lived a protected existence away from the outside "normal" world and obviously there would be times when we rebelled! When I was 15 a group of us decided we would set dares for each other. One girl got drunk on vodka and another stole a lip gloss from Woolworths. Mine was to runaway and see how far I could get before they caught me. My friends had a whip round and raised about £13. So on a summer evening after dinner I called a taxi and walked to the back entrance of the School. Now, I knew from previous attempts by girls to run away that the first thing the staff would do would be to ring the local train station, Alton, to ask if I had been there. With this in mind I asked the taxi to take me to Bentley Station, which was the next stop along the journey to Waterloo. I knew the route really well as at times, instead of driving me back at the beginning of term my Dad would take me by train from Leicester to St Pancras. From there we would catch a cab across to Waterloo where we would be met by School staff who would take over and accompany any students that were returning by train to back to Treloars. And so from Bentley Station I boarded the train to Waterloo with no further plan in mind, all the time expecting to get caught when I got off the train and escorted back to Treloars. No one was waiting. Now the sensible thing to do would be to get on a train back to Alton, take a taxi back to Treloars and be back before anyone noticed. I could hold my head high having taken the dare and succeed not to get caught.

No, that isn't what I did.

In fact I did the only thing I really knew how to do and that was to take a cab to St Pancras Station. I'm 15 and travelling across London alone at night. I had no luggage with me and when the taxi driver asked me where I was going, I said I was going home to Leicester as I had been staying with friends in London. He asked why I didn't have any luggage and I can't remember what excuse I gave but he didn't ask any more questions. Once at St Pancras I checked the price of a ticket to Leicester and had just enough left from my £13. I had absolutely no idea what I was going to do next but I boarded the train.

Now remember we didn't have mobile phones so there were no texts from my friends updating me on the panic that was ensuing amongst the Treloars staff. Once they realised I was missing they had contacted my parents and questioned my friends. Eventually they confessed but denied they had anything to do with it and that it was all my idea!! I can't blame them really. Well, I was for the high jump so no point taking anyone else down with me I suppose.

I got off the train at Leicester Station and it would have been about 11.30pm I think. I didn't know what I was going to do but I didn't have to make any more decisions because Dad was standing there waiting for me. You have no idea how relieved I was. Parents were not at all happy with me. They made that quite clear and so I was dutifully returned a few days later. Many years later they confessed that actually they were really quite proud of my achievement! Mum said she would have done the same thing, couldn't back down and once the journey started would have to of just kept going. These days I would never have the confidence to go that distance alone at night, but then we didn't really know about all the dangers out there in the big world because we were protected by Treloars for most of the time.

The current Lord Mayor of London would visit us once a year. We had to be on our very best behaviour on that day. Leading up to the day our uniforms were checked and if any were looking worn or shabby, or a little outgrown then it would be replaced with a new one which had to be saved for the special visit. Cutlery was polished, floors were scrubbed and windows all gleaming! He would come to each classroom and observe. Of course we rehearsed what he would see. Prepped by teachers to put a hand up and ask a question that we already knew the answer to because we had practised it days before. He would watch, smile and move on to the next classroom, totally unaware, I'm sure that it was all just for his benefit!

I loved the sport that Treloars offered me. My favourite was swimming. I think all those years of crutches use gave me the upper body strength to be good enough to compete and yearly took part in the Stoke Mandeville Junior Games. Dr Ludwig Guttman was a respected Jewish neurosurgeon who had fled his homeland of Germany in 1939. In 1944 he was asked by the British Government to open a Spinal Injuries Unit at Stoke Mandeville. On July 29th 1948 which was the day of the Opening Ceremony of the London 1948 Olympic Games, a competition for wheelchair athletes took place at Stoke Mandeville. Dr Guttman organised 14 men and two women to take place in an archery tournament. By the following year Stoke Mandeville hosted six teams competing in Wheelchair Netball and over the years more teams and more sports were added. And so today we have the Paralympics all thanks to the man who recognised the value of sport to the disabled and those rehabilitating from a disability. In 2012 the BBC broadcast a drama titled "The best of men" portraying

Ludwig Guttman's years as a doctor at Stoke Mandeville Hospital where he treats wounded British soldiers with spinal injuries. When he arrives at the hospital the patients are sedated and kept immobilised and his mission is to prove to the other staff that mobility really is the best route to recovery. The Stoke Mandeville Junior games that I took part in from 1972 weren't like the Olympics or even Paralympics where you competed in your own particular specialised area whatever that may be. No, we were all rounder's. Wheelchair Dash, Shot Put, Javelin, Basketball, Table Tennis, Wheelchair Slalom. You name it and I took part. We were placed in categories according to disability. In simple terms this meant that if your legs didn't work but both arms did you would be Grade 3, Sight impairment Grade 2, etc. On one visit to Stoke Mandeville I met a man who examined me to make sure I was in the correct category. That man was "Professor" Ludwig Guttman. He was a great man of foresight who I feel extremely privileged to have met.

I learnt to canoe at Treloars. We once did a demonstration at Crystal Palace to show how disability in sport could be so versatile and wasn't just about swimming and wheelchair racing and my party piece was to make it appear that I was under water holding my breath. With my parents in the spectator's seats watching, I paddled my canoe into the middle of the pool and rolled upside down. Our instructor announced to the spectators that I was "perfectly fine" when after more than a minute I hadn't reappeared. Mum was panicking. Although I can hold my breath for quite a while, that wasn't the case. On rolling under the water, the spray deck was pulled off and I swam under the boat so my head was inside the cockpit, breathing the trapped air inside. After counting to just over sixty seconds I resurfaced to the applause. At another exhibition at a University somewhere, we were supposed to all roll over into the water again, but the water was so cold I didn't do it. I just sat in mine and waited to be chastised by Mrs Bell while all my teammates did as they were told. I couldn't get the hang of full Eskimo rolls where you turn the boat upside down then back upright again doing a full 360 degree movement. I don't think my hips were strong enough but I had good upper body strength from all the swimming. Whilst taking part in the Duke of Edinburgh Awards Scheme I also canoed eleven and a half miles along the River Arun. Exhausting but satisfying. In a canoe everyone is equal!! No crutches, no wheelchair and no callipers.

The track events consisted mainly of Wheelchair racing. This was known as Wheelchair Dash. Field events were archery, precision and distance javelin, shot put and discus. Horse riding was another popular pastime at Treloars. Before going there my parents used to take me to a riding school for the disabled in Fleckney, Leicestershire. I rode a pony called Peanuts but if a peanut wasn't available then Minty was my next choice.

My dad would lift me and place me on the pony but at Treloars it wasn't a case of being lifted. At the riding school in Medstead, which was a couple of miles away from Treloars, there was a dip where the pony would stand while we would either walk or wheel along a platform so that the horse was at our seat height. Then we could simply transfer across, a bit like getting into a car. Again, being on a horse gave a sense of equality like canoeing. No mobility aids required once on the horse. These days I get that same feeling from driving a car. Once in the car, no one else can see the disability.

After leaving Treloars I continued with my competitive swimming and joined a Nottingham Club. I took part in the Senior Games and passed the selection for the 1984 Los Angeles Paralympics. I didn't continue and gave up the training in 1982 when I married for the first time.

Apart from sport my other big interest was boys! Thanks to Lord Mayor Treloar and his foresight back in 1907 and then building a boys School close by in Froyle, this was made all the more easier for me. Just a short taxi ride away! We became very good at inventing reasons to visit them or for them to visit us. Some of us signed up to attend a folk group which entailed getting out into the town on a weekday evening. Convincing teachers that we were interested in subjects that were only available at the boys school so we would have to go there. Sneaking out in the evenings to go to meet up there was fun. I wasn't the only one though I must say, although I often got the blame for instigating it. Yes I was gated more times than I can remember but it was all part of the excitement. "Gated" was the equivalent of "Grounded" that parents punish their children with. So called because it we were forbidden to go out of the school gates for the duration of the punishment. The junior house matrons were lovely and not that much older than us and once when I was gated I smuggled my boyfriend into the house matrons flat at the bottom of the pink corridor with their help. Of course I got caught when for some reason the Deputy Head, Mr Cocksedge decided he needed to inspect the flat. Maybe someone grassed me up or maybe I wasn't as good at concealing my boyfriend as I thought. Double Gated! One day my friend Sally and I thought it would be good fun to take ourselves to the family planning clinic and ask for the pill. We thought it would be a really grown up thing to

54

do, as we had just turned 16. I was asked some question about whether I had a boyfriend and had we had sex. Yes I declared proudly. After being examined the nurse declared me to be "hymen intact" (still a virgin) and refused me the pill. She knew I was lying. Many years later, in 2015, when I returned to Treloars for a reunion my friend Janet and I discovered they had put condom machines in the toilets. Oh how times have changed.

Treloars taught me independence and sport which is good because academically I can't say I was much of an achiever. It also made us realise that if we wanted to be accepted in society when we left Treloars, then we would need to make ourselves as "normal" as possible. Make the disability, whatever it was, invisible. Not like today where we are encouraged to be ourselves no matter what that is. These were different times. No Equality Act or even Disability Discrimination Act. No, we were expected to fit in to "normal world" even though that meant numerous limitations. We could not expect "normal world" to accept us for whom and what we were.

The main thing I struggled with wasn't so much the separation from home. It was the isolation on returning home. Back and forth every couple of months you don't build up any friendships or relationships. You get home and everyone is moving on with their lives and every time it was like moving to a new house or school and a feeling of not really fitting in or belonging. On leaving I was given the opportunity to attend Hereward College in Coventry for disabled students. I went for the interview which included an overnight stay. I decided it wasn't for me. I needed to go home and somehow break the isolation and make it work.

Instead I enrolled at Hinckley College of Further Education in Leicestershire to do an Ordinary National Diploma in Business Studies. The course lasted two years and at least I could live back at home again amongst the "non disabled"

More moves

1974 – 1978

Of all the houses I lived in as a child my favourite was one on Hinckley Road, Leicester Forest East. From 1961 to 1978, when I left Treloars, we had lived in six houses. Six house moves and four Schools. My parents had been given a grant by Leicestershire County Council to convert part of the downstairs for me and so the old dining room became a bedroom with en-suite shower and toilet. Mum had decided by the time I became a teenager clambering up stairs on all fours and scrambling back down again head first was becoming a little undignified and not at all ladylike. I loved my room with its purple wallpaper and kidney shaped dressing table with a purple curtain hiding the drawers. Whenever I came home from Treloars I would lie on my bed late at night listening to Radio Luxemburg. Radio Luxembourg was transmitted into the UK from Luxembourg by a long wave frequency. It was a popular choice as an alternative to the BBC. But its adverts were annoying. Particularly when you were trying to record your favourite songs on your cassette recorder and the song would be cut off before the end for an advert break.

For a long time the BBC had the monopoly on UK radio transmissions but in 1973 new legislation allowed independent radio stations to broadcast funded by advertising sales.

Every time I came home it was hard to rekindle friendships. It was so difficult to re-connect. Social media would have made that so much easier. Just a quick status update on my Facebook wall to announce "Hey, I'm back at home again" But for me, by the time I could make any contact it was time to go back. If I'm honest, I was little lonely when at home. Chris used to bring his mates round and they would play poker and three card brag while mum and dad were out at work. I had some friends and I would write to them from school to let them know I was coming back. They would come round so we could catch up. Often they would be doing things that it was impossible for me such as roller skating or playing tennis perhaps. I could always sense the embarrassment when they made excuses about what they were doing. I guess they didn't want to leave me out and that was ok because I knew that as soon as I got back to Treloars, there was no such awkwardness. But it wasn't until I left Treloars for good and started college that I could make any real friendships in Leicester.

There was a wall outside the front of our house and I would spend hours just sitting there watching the world go by. Sometimes people would stop and talk to me. It seems odd now, but to me it was just a way of passing the time.

Chris had a friend called Bernie who was a couple of years older than him. Bernie had his own flat down the road and it was always full of teenagers who liked to hang out with Bernie. Bernie told us that he had an identical twin and that following an argument with his parents he had moved out. It had been weeks before his parents noticed he wasn't there. His twin covered for him. He worked for BT but was also a mechanic and his flat always smelt of petrol and oil. I was in Bernie's flat on the 16th August 1977 when we heard the news Elvis Presley had died. I went home and put Radio Luxembourg on in my bedroom. DJ Tony Prince just kept saying over and over again "The King is dead"

In my last year at Treloars we moved again. This time the move was to a three story house in the village of Desford, in Leicestershire. This house had three floors, but my bedroom was on the ground floor and there was a downstairs bathroom with toilet off the hallway. There was a living room and a dining room too but when dad decided he wanted to work from home, they needed my room to make into the dining room as he had taken the original one as his office. And so I was moved onto the second floor. Dad sold it to me by saying it was more "Normal" to have a bedroom upstairs. I had to learn to walk up the stairs by putting my right crutch in my left hand and using the banister to haul myself up. One day mum said she wondered why she kept seeing black marks on the wall. It was my crutch dragging along it!

Chris was working at Ross's on the M1 (later to become Welcome Break) and if he was on the early shift he needed to get up at 6am. Now don't ask me why because I have no idea, but I would set my alarm to wake me up and this was at a time when my bedroom was still on the ground floor and climb up two flights of stairs where his bedroom was on the third floor to wake him. Then I would go back down the same stairs to the kitchen and make him a cup of tea. If he didn't appear I would go back up again and re wake him, wait for a couple of minutes to be sure he was awake, then go back down again. As soon as I heard the front door close I would go back to sleep. Was it an attempt to be useful? Did I need his approval? Who knows because I don't? I do remember that it didn't seem like a chore at the time. I have no idea why we needed such a big house but I can only imagine it was a status thing. We can afford it so we are buying it maybe. My dad's business was very successful so why not, if you can afford it. I know I would.

Mum and I would fall out quite a lot after I returned from Treloars. It was hard adjusting to life within a family again after long months away. We argued about so many things and I would walk out the house. I would walk to the park and just sit there for hours, waiting for her or dad to come and look for me. Sometimes dad came to find me then we would go back to the house and mum would say "So you've finished sulking then" I don't really know what the arguments were about. Dad once said that he thought it was because me and mum were too much alike. If I was upset or annoyed by anything mum would say, "Watch out, she's having one of her traumas again" That would make me laugh and everything would be ok again. I was just a stroppy teenager I guess.

One thing I hated and still do is eating on my own. I hated it if they had dinner before I got home and I had to reheat mine and sit alone in the kitchen. We didn't have the luxury of portable TV's in the kitchen in those days. I wonder whether it was because I was so used the eating meals in a dining room full of students and teachers or even on a hospital ward.

Europa Lodge, home to the stars!

1977-1979

Whilst studying for my diploma in Business studies at Hinckley College, I persuaded the manager at my local pub to give me a job. The Europa Lodge was a "Motel" on the A47 close to junction 21 of the M1. My friends and I had adopted this as a temporary local while The Red Cow just down the road was being refurbished. After the refurbishment was complete we would flit between the two as this was just within my scale of walking distances. According to Google Maps this is a distance of half a mile and should take about 10 minutes. I'm pretty sure it took me longer than that, but it was manageable, that's the important thing. Well this job wasn't much but it gave me a bit of spending money. I typed the menus for the evening meals and any other small bits of typing that were required from time to time. This was 1979 and I would sit at the back of reception using their manual typewriter to type "The menu of the Day" Although Electric typewriters were easier and more popular this hotel didn't have one. Word processors hadn't been invented and we were a long way from computers so it was a slow process. So there I would sit, "Clickety clacking" away with my trusty bottle of Tipex correcting fluid nearby.

The Assistant Manager was a man called Mark and he had the idea that he wanted to make this hotel into something really trendy that celebrities would want to stay at when performing in Leicester. Its close proximity to the M1 made it ideal. This is how I came by my infamous Debbie Harry story. Blondie were booked to play at De Montfort Hall and her management team had requested she was booked into a Suite. Unfortunately for Mark, Europa Lodge didn't have a Suite but it did have a conference room. Mark came up with the idea of making the conference room look like a bedroom suite but he was lacking a 3 piece suit which was necessary if he was going to pull this off. At home, our dining room had a brown, corded one and I asked mum if the hotel could borrow it. Yes, as long as they collected it and returned it she said. Mark got me tickets for the concert as a thank you for saving his reputation and I went with my friend Sally to the show. When the suite was returned to us at home when it was not longer needed, it had a cigarette burn. My story always begins with "Have I ever told you about the time Debbie Harry put a cigarette burn in my mum's sofa?" Now of course I have no idea how it got there, it could have been anyone and was more likely to have happened when it was in transit by the delivery drivers. We will never know.

Ian Dury and the Blockheads also stayed there and in the bar my friends and I used to chat to the roadies. I managed to get on the guest list to the concert which was also at De Montfort Hall. I went with Chris. After the show, one of the roadies came and asked if we would like to meet Ian. Off we went back stage and were introduced to him, along with a guy called Graham who was there with his friend. Graham was blind and I guess we were selected as, like Ian Dury, we had disabilities. Ian gave us both a T-shirt and signed them. On Graham's shirt he wrote in black marker pen "Graham is a fucking twat" Graham asked him what he had written and Ian told him. "I can't wear that to the blind school" was Graham's shocked response. To which Ian's quick reply was "It's ok, no one will see it" Mine said "Steph is a nonce" I didn't know what that meant so Ian explained that it meant someone who is put in prison for doing naughty things to children. Odd sense of humour, but a lovely man nevertheless. The roadies told me that Ian would be approached all the time by women who wanted to have sex with a "ripple" (cockney rhyming slang for cripple)

On the subject of celebrities I have met, Danny La Rue had an apartment at Royal Palm in

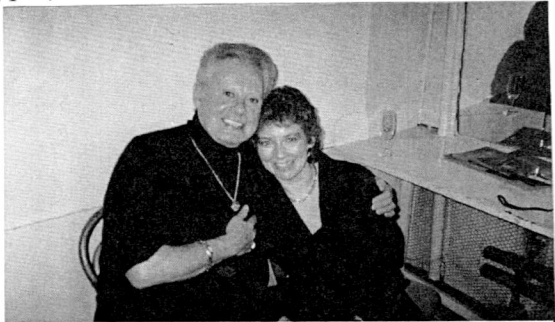

The late, great, fabulous Danny La Rue and me, Leeds 1989

Tenerife where my parents lived in the 1980s. He was a lovely man and I met him a few times. In fact I went to his 60th birthday party that he held at a bar called "Georges" in Los Cristianos. He used to sit by the swimming pool chatting with whoever stopped to speak. Amazing that people recognised him in his bathing attire and without his famous frocks and make-up. He invited me to his show in Leeds. My friend Karen and I arrived a little late and were shown to our seats, quite high up "in the gods" as they say. During the interval we were approached by a man who said "Danny is asking where you are, you are meant to be in a "box" near the stage. And so we watched the rest of the show like royalty.

During his act he was dressed as Joan Collins. "Joan" said that her sister Jackie writes books and her friend Jennifer over in Tenerife likes to read them. It was nice. He had personalised his act for my benefit, Jennifer being my mum of course. He was a lovely man.

Another claim to fame was meeting Peter Noon of Herman's Hermits when he came to open our annual Christmas Fayre. I was selling lavender bags that we had made and his wife bought some from me.

During those days of Europa Lodge I was in there one night with friends and it was packed out. It always was during the days of the Red Cow being out of action. The local football team were called "Racing Green" and they had a match that day against a team from Braunstone. I tried to squeeze past the Braunstone lads to get out and one of them said "Move out the way, let this cripple past" One of our local boys took great offence at this and a fight broke out in the bar which then spilled out into the car park. The Police were called and one of the Police Officers came over to where I was sitting on a wall watching. He asked me if I had been involved at all and my friend spoke up for me and said "No, she wasn't" I think it was just an excuse for a punch up between two rival teams and I was used as the justification for it. On another occasion I was there when I heard someone refer to me as K9 – the metal dog from Dr Who. Quite upsetting as this was a person I had thought of as a friend. They didn't know at the time I was within hearing distance but I was very wary of them after that.

Management at Europa Lodge decided to go even more upmarket and on a Friday night would transform the dining room into a nightclub. I again persuaded them to give me the job as receptionist and would sit on my bar stool signing people in and issuing membership cards. The Club Copacabana didn't last long. It was expensive for them to run and they didn't have the right licence for late night drinking.

I finished working at the Europa Lodge when I was admitted to hospital for further surgery. Whilst I'd been away they had replaced me!

The incident with the Solicitors Milk

1979

My next temporary job was during the summer holidays of 1979. My parents persuaded their friend David Inman, to give me a job in his one man Solicitors practice in Hinckley, Leicestershire. I was 17 and learning to drive but had not yet passed my test. It was a made up "Office Junior" position and if anyone reading this has ever had a "temporary office junior position" you will know exactly what that really means. "Dogsbody and tea maker" The office was in an old converted terraced house on the second floor. Downstairs was occupied by a small firm of Chartered Accountants and as I looked at the steep flight of stairs in front of me I wished they had given me a job instead.

On my first day I met Mr Inman's secretary Mary. She wasn't what you would call friendly and welcoming. Mary eyed me up and couldn't exactly hide the fact that David had not prepared her. It was clear she did not want this intrusion. She was important to David. She was his sole employee. She certainly didn't want some bright eyed, all knowing, 17yr old college student in the way. Not only that, but a 17 yr old with obvious physical limitations. I'd just climbed up a steep flight of stairs and was red faced, and a little out of breath and desperately wanted to sit down. Whenever I was with Mum and we were confronted by stairs, she would take one crutch so that I could hold onto the banister with one hand and use it as leverage. Sometimes when reaching the top she would forget and carry on walking, leaving me stranded at the top of the stairs. Anyway, Mary didn't have time for me to rest. She wasn't having any of that. She sent me out to buy milk as my first task.

Ok....I had never had to buy a pint of milk before. At home ours was always delivered by a milkman but if we did run out, Mum would go to the Co-Op and buy a bottle. No way was I going to ask Mary where to get if from. She wasn't going to have that satisfaction. So I went back down the stairs and walked towards the town. The only place I could think of would be the Co-Op on Castle Street. It was one of those big Co-Ops that sold everything from beds to clothes and more importantly to me, milk. It was about 480 metres or 1580 feet from David's office. If you have ever had to use crutches, for whatever reason, you will appreciate the task ahead of me. Now Mary could have completed the whole task in less than 15 minutes, there and back. It took me 20 minutes just to get to the shop. Back in the 1970's 95% of milk was sold in glass bottles. No lightweight plastic or Tetra Paks. It's a good job I didn't drop the blasted thing on the way back. The bottle was in a paper bag as plastic carrier bags weren't available back then. I had to keep my hand at the end of the handle on the crutch as far from the metal stick part to prevent it from smashing as I swung my way back to the office. .

So there we are. I'm on crutches and have walked about thirty minutes to buy a bottle of milk and then had to struggle thirty minutes back again and up the stairs back to the office. I was knackered.

Smug Mary looked up from her typing and said "Oh that took you a long time; I thought you weren't coming back". If it hadn't been for the fact I was in desperate need of tea I'd have smashed that bottle over her head. Of course she did it deliberately. Mary did not like sharing Mr Inman.

I worked there throughout the summer of 1979 before going back to college and was paid £25 a week.

Driving

It seemed imperative to me that I learnt to drive as soon as possible. By August 1978, the year I could apply for my Provisional Licence we were living in Desford which was a bus ride away from my friends in Leicester Forest East and Kirby Muxloe. I relied heavily on lifts from dad or Chris but if they weren't available it was public transport. And buses didn't have those lifts on like they do today. It was a case of just climbing the steps and holding the bus up.

Mum bought a yellow mini and we had hand controls fitted. If you don't know about hand controls and how they operate let me try to explain. There is a connecting rod that is attached to the brake and another rod attached to the accelerator. They meet at a bar just below the steering wheel. You push the bar down to brake and pull it up to accelerate. Simple! This does mean that they only work on automatic cars as one hand is braking and accelerating and the other one is steering. Not a good idea to take your hand of the steering wheel every time you need to change gears. The controls were fitted and my licence arrived. We found a driving instructor who was prepared to take the risk of teaching me in the mini. He would have had dual controls if we were in a driving school car so I can only say thank you to that man for putting his life in my hands.

My lessons began in March 1979 and took place in Hinckley, Leicestershire. The winter of 1978 / 79 had been a particularly harsh one. It was named "The Winter of Discontent" because of the widespread strikes in the public sector but many thought that name that should also apply to the weather. Temperatures throughout that winter rarely moved above zero and snow and blizzards were dominant. The knock on effect for learner drivers was that this meant a backlog. Hundred of tests were cancelled through the winter months and the average waiting time for one was six months. With this is mind my instructor told me to apply after only a couple of lessons. When test day arrived I was confident that this was going to be the day that I was truly free. In a car no one can see your disabled. Driving a car makes you equal. I would be able to get anywhere I wanted without the struggle of buses and trains. I could drive myself and do what I pleased in my proper "normal" car. The lessons cost £5 an hour. They would have been £7 but because I was in my own car and using my own petrol he reduced the fee. A test in 1979 cost £25 and there was no theory test just the practical with the examiner asking some questions about the Highway Code when you got back to the test station. They would then tell you if you had passed or failed. Rumour was that if the examiner asked you questions about driving on the motorway as part of your Highway Code knowledge, then you knew you had passed before he had the chance to tell you.

In Britain throughout the 60's and 70's the NHS provided "Invalid Carriages" as a low-cost vehicle to aid the mobility of people with disabilities. These vehicles were bright blue and had three wheels. They were also very lightweight and often blew over in the wind or tip. They were only designed to carry one person and they had the nickname "Noddy Cars" because of how they looked. If you had one you needed four or five driving lessons and then you could be independent. I didn't have one at Treloars, I don't think I was old enough but I knew those that did. To be honest I wouldn't have wanted one. Who wants to go out and about looking like that? I was barely tolerating a wheelchair but to have a big blue carriage was a step too far! Image is important isn't it? Independence is one things but that was just too much!. Even our Headmistress at Treloars, Miss Anderson had one. She would drive around Florence Treloars grounds with her little dog on a lead running alongside her. Even though it was illegal to carry passengers, there was only one seat, they often did. With the passenger sitting on the floor! Not surprising that they kept tipping over!

Anyway, I failed at first attempt. The examiner was a Mr Foster. He wore a navy raincoat and had dark glasses. I thought he looked quite sinister. I was devastated but then not many people pass at first attempt do they? I know my mum didn't. He said "I'm sorry Miss Pollock, you have not yet reached the standard required" and handed me my failure notice.

Mum set about getting me a second test. You had to wait one calendar month before you could try again and the waiting list was still over six months long. Exactly 1 month later she put me on a cancellation list. In May I got a cancellation and went for attempt number two. I was going to pass this time because everyone passed by the second test didn't they?

Again Mr Foster got into the car. Again Mr Foster failed me. Oh the shame. two failures! No one I knew of failed twice. The first failure had been approaching junctions too quickly. The second was for approaching junctions too slowly.

Never mind, give it a month and try for another cancellation. When Mr Foster got into my car in July I was ready for him. I was going to show him I could drive. "I'm sorry Miss Pollock you've not quite reached the standard required" No, not again. What was wrong with me? My instructor said I could drive as well as anyone he had ever taught and yet at the test, the crucial moment, I seemed to lose it. My dad had been known to fall asleep once or twice when I had driven him around while practising so I couldn't be that bad. Dad had a theory that I struggled a bit because I'd never ridden a bike so had never developed any road sense. I also blame that theory for the fact I have no sense of direction either. If it's not mapped out in front of me, I'm lost. Thank heavens for Sat Navs!

And so it came to be that on 27th September 1979 I set of for test number four

Mr Foster got into my car and smiled for the first time at me. It was like we were old friends. Mum had said to me, "This time just think sod it, and go for it" I went for it. I drove as if I had been doing it for years. I found the confidence. Maybe it was because he had smiled at me.

He barely looked at his paper as we did reversing round corners, emergency stops, three point turns. As it was an automatic I wasn't required to do a hill start though. Mr Foster shook my hand when he got out of the car. I had done it. Four tests in six months and just past my 18th Birthday I got there.

Our house had three storeys and if you stood in Chris's bedroom and looked out of the window you could see right down Peckleton Lane towards the A47. This was our return route from Hinckley Test Centre. Mum and dad where standing in that window with a pair of binoculars looking for me. They were desperate to see if the L Plates had been removed. No mobile phones back then to ring or text the news. No, they had to wait for our return. Now for some reason and I don't really remember why, my instructor drove me home. He said it was something to do with the insurance but maybe it was because he thought I would crash the car because of all the excitement of finally doing it. They saw that little yellow mini coming down the road, L Plates still on and my Instructor driving it. But as soon as they saw my face they knew. They both had tears. Pride? More like relief I expect. Dad and Chris could hang up their taxi hats.

In 1977 Lord Sterling of Plaistow created a charitable organisation called Motability. It was designed to assist disabled drivers to afford cars to suit their needs. The way it worked was this. You could go to an authorised car dealer and select a car to suit your needs as long as you were receiving the Mobility Allowance. You would then sign over the Mobility Allowance and keep the car for three years. And then when the three years were up you handed it back and started again. Insurance was provided as was breakdown cover but the hand controls had to be self financed. There was never any worry about MOT's as you never kept the car longer than three years. No road tax to pay either as disabled drivers are exempt. The choice of cars was limited as were the choice of colours but for many it was the only affordable way to get a car. The reason I am writing this in the past tense is not because the scheme no longer exists but that this was the deal when I got my first one in 1979. It was a brown Mini. I loved it.

Over the years the rules kept changing. For a period of time you could only have Red, White or Blue. They ruled for some time that you could only do 10,000 miles a year and any mileage above that you were charged for. Many of the cars were available with no down payment such as my mini, but if you wanted a bigger better car you would be required to pay an initial deposit. After time the cost of the hand controls was included which was a big help as I was paying around £450 every three years and they always went back with the car. You couldn't transfer them from one car to another even if it was the same make as car designs are constantly changing and they wouldn't have fitted properly. It never once occurred to me to ask for them back and sell them second hand to someone else. When Attendance and Mobility Allowance were combined to make the Disability Living Allowance (and now PIP - Personal Independence Payment) the qualifying rule was that you must be on the Higher Rate Component of the mobility component.

In 2018 Motability came in for some criticism when the National Audit Office discovered that the boss of Motability, this charitable organisation, was in line for a £2.2 million bonus by 2022. In December 2018 he resigned. There was also an investigation into why Motability was stockpiling £2.4 billion in cash and assets. Motability is accountable for about 10% of all new cars bought in the UK. Not bad for a charity. The NAO accused Motability of charging customers £390 million more than was required since 2008.

I had a couple of gaps as a Motability customer. In 1982 when the mini was due to be returned and I was married to my first husband, Eamon (more about him later) we decided we needed the money instead and didn't order a new one. When I say "we" I'm not sure I was truly happy with that decision. He found me a cheap car to drive and I've no idea where we got the hand controls from but it served a purpose. Insurance was an issue back then when you you're not using the Motability Scheme. Apparently disabled drivers are risky. I found a company though that was a "Disabled Drivers Specialist" called Chartwell. Eventually that little white car, whatever it was, gave up and the wheel fell off when I was driving one day.

My next car was bought from the son of one of my dad's clients. It was a Daf 66 which was a variomatic rather than automatic. My brother joked that it ran on an elastic band. Dad ordered the hand controls mail order and fitted them himself. One day I was out driving and suddenly something went wrong. They had worked their way loose somehow and stopped working. Fortunately one of my brother's mates just happened to be driving by and stopped. He fixed them with a safety pin so I could get home. The Daf however didn't last long either. This was in the days when you needed a choke to start the car in cold weather and first the choke broke and then the radiator kept overheating. After so many times of coming out to rescue me, mum said "Right, that's enough. You're going back to Motability. She took me to the Vauxhall Dealer but he said we might be better off taking out a finance plan to purchase the car and using the Mobility Allowance to cover the payments. I had a Suzuki Alto in a fabulous metallic blue for seven years.

In 1992 I went back to Motability to trade in the Suzuki and order a new car. Well I tried to. In the 90's there weren't so many Motability car dealers in Leicester. Now they are everywhere. This is how I ended up at Swithland Motors. I ordered my car from a lady called Angela who was the sales assistant and was the dealers "Motability Expert" She assured me that my car would only take about eight weeks and then I would be driving away in my brand new shiny red Rover Metro. Several months passed by and no sign of my car. Every time I rang Angela gave me phrases like "Production issues" "Not our fault" "Out of our hands" but she always assured me that my car was "Imminent". Eventually I cancelled my order and went elsewhere. A short time later Swithland Motors hit the news. In 1993 Swithland Motors collapsed owing £15 million and the Directors were imprisoned for false accounting, bogus transactions, and falsified documents. They were accused of creating "Ingenious Scams" to deceive bankers, Investors, Finance Companies and Auditors. On one occasion when the Auditors were due to visit the owners entered the details of all the staffs cars onto their books and parked them on the forecourt to make it look like they had more stock than they actually did. I've no idea whether my Metro was ever ordered in the first place but I suspect probably not.

I stayed with Motability after that until 2018 when I needed to make some cutbacks and started looking at ways to save money. It was then I did the sums. The mobility component of PIP in 2018 was £59.75 a week. Over three years that's £9321 that I was giving them and then handing the car back. Ok so I know I get peace of mind driving a brand new car and am covered with insurance and breakdown cover in that price but it still seemed a lot to me. Not surprising that they are making so much money. Plus I was finding it increasingly difficult getting in and out of the car. I had a Skoda Yeti by this time. I looked at Wheelchair Adapted Vehicles (WAV) on Motability but the Initial Deposit required was way out of my price range.

After a lot of discussion, researching and comparing notes with my Trelorian friends I opted out of Motability again and went for private finance on a Renault Master with an electric tail lift. It cost about £300 to put the hand controls on (yes they have come down in price) and we put the insurance in Graham's name (more about him later) because under Motability Insurance one of their terms was that I wouldn't earn any No Claims Bonus. Adding up the cost of repayments to the finance company, insurance, breakdown cover the Mobility component of PIP was covering it all with a little left over towards yearly MOT and Servicing.

Yes it's a big vehicle for someone who is only 4ft 8" but I can get in and out pain free with ease and feel like I'm king of the road when I'm driving

Proper job!
1979

Straight from leaving College 1979 I had to register at the Job Centre in order to be able to claim "Dole" money. They told me I would need a green card to prove to prospective employers that I was truly disabled and disadvantaged in finding work. I expect this was not so much to make employers feel sorry for me but more to fulfil their quota of 1 "Registered Disabled" person per 100 employees. Because I lived more than four miles out of the city (we were living in Desford by then) I was permitted to sign on by post. Every two weeks I would receive a form in the post to sign and have witnessed, then post it back and the Giro would arrive on a Thursday.

My first proper job didn't come about until 1980. When I left college my mother took me into Leicester and I tried registering at several agencies. Not an easy task. Yes they agreed to put me on the books but made it clear that options were restricted for me. On one of these outings we bumped into a friend of Mum's called Anne. Mum said we were looking for work for me and Anne told us of a vacancy at the Insurance Brokers where she worked. So I went for the interview at Bankarts on Charles Street in Leicester. They must have been way ahead of the game because they said I could have a parking permit in the nearby NCP that they would pay for to make things easier - I think you would call it a "Reasonable Adjustment" today. Remember, no wheelchair in those days and it was quite a walk for me to get to the Office but at least they had a lift in the building. Then after being offered the job Mum took me to C&A on the corner of Charles Street and Humberstone Gate and got me kitted out with a whole wardrobe of what she called "Office Suitable Attire"

At Bankarts I saw my first computer. It was as big as four fridge freezers joined together!!

I had a few health problems over the next couple of years with a recurring ulcer on my ankle. It stemmed from the plastic cosmetic callipers that rubbed on my skin. With no sensation you can't tell that you are causing harm. I couldn't walk without the callipers and I couldn't wear the callipers with the ulcer problem. After a period of time off sick from work I returned using my wheelchair. Oh god that was so much easier!! Once again Mr Stoyle came to my rescue. He decided to take a piece of skin from my thigh, where the circulation and skin was healthier, and pack it into the ulcer in my ankle. It worked and as soon as the wound healed I returned to work on crutches. My boss called me into his office to say he hoped that I was now healing well, but that he thought I should come to work in my wheelchair in future. Now I know that I said it was easier, like getting from car park to office etc, but I was proud and programmed to believe that crutches are best and wheelchairs make you fat and lazy. I refused and shortly after was made redundant. Coincidence?!

I tried again to get a job but the opportunities just weren't there. Unemployment was pretty high in the 1980's and to be disabled made it virtually impossible unless you knew someone, who knew someone that was prepared to take a chance. I went for an interview at an optician in Leicester. I decided to be brave and at the end when he asked the question "Is there anything you would like to ask me?" I said "Will my disability affect your decision as to whether to offer me the job?" Reply…. "Well yes obviously" I didn't get the job and neither would I have accepted it.

A friend of mine, from Treloar days, Janet, told me that after leaving school she went for an interview at a bank. The interviewer told her they couldn't offer her the job as her face would put people off as she looked a little different. She has a brittle bone condition

Osteogenesis Imperfecta and people with this condition have characteristically an "owl like" face appearance. By no means unattractive. This is merely a symptom of her disability. It is shocking to think how small minded employers were permitted to be before the introduction of the Disability Discrimination Act 1995

In the 1980's Leicester City Council had a scheme where they would advertise vacancies but you could only apply if you were "Registered Disabled" I applied for one and was interviewed. Didn't get offered it until their first choice turned them down. I declined it as it at the Shopmobility Office in an NCP in Leicester City Centre and some of the time I would be working alone. Alone, in a car park didn't appeal to me.

By 1995 things changed. The Disability Discrimination Act was introduced

Disabled persons looking for work could be guaranteed an interview providing they covered the essential criteria for the role. This meant we could no longer be paper sifted out but could be offered a slightly better chance of at least getting an interview. The Act also meant that employers would be able to ask for help from the Government in making reasonable adjustments if the disabled person was the most suitable for the position, but that facilities would prevent the job being offered.

In 1986 I was summoned for Jury Service. I was really looking forward to it strangely enough. Maybe two weeks away from work and doing something interesting.

I arrived at the Court on the first day and sat in the room along with all the others that had been summoned. We were told what would be expected of us by a Court Usher but that we probably wouldn't be needed that first day as there was an ongoing case that was just coming to its conclusion so it would be more likely the next day when we would be called. I returned the second day and we were taken into the court to wait being sworn in. I wasn't selected so made my way back to the waiting room. At this point the Court Usher came to speak to me. He apologised. He said "I have just been advised by the judge that we shouldn't really have called you. We didn't realise how difficult it would be for you to serve due to your mobility problems" Presumably being in the court was the first time a Judge had spotted me amongst the rest. I was told to go home as they wouldn't need me. I protested. I said it wasn't a problem and that I could perfectly manage, but he wasn't having any of it so my Jury Service ended after just two days.

In 1999 I applied for a part-time switchboard position at Leicester General Hospital. I passed the telephone task and the face to face interview and received a phone call the next day saying I came top of all the interviewees and they wished to offer me a position. However, before they could commence my employment there were certain issues that they needed to address. I could have a parking space with my name on, then if I walked along the corridor to the switch room they would have a wheelchair in situ for me to use. The wheelchair was provided by Access to Work. Yes sounds good. You may wonder why they did not place the wheelchair by the door from the car park. They were afraid the porters would take it and use it for patients!! Good point - it was a hospital after all. By this time I was using a wheelchair more and more and only used the crutches when necessary.

Second adjustment was that there was a step inside the room. They needed to make it ramped. Thirdly, the fire exit at the rear of the room was rough ground. They wanted to slab it to make is wheelchair friendly. Fourthly and major issue of all…. There was a large 6ft tall board inside the room that was a control panel for the fire alarms in and around the hospital.   The role of the switchboard operator was to monitor this board and if an alarm activated, switch the button off on the board and call the Fire Brigade! Every Saturday afternoons I would be sole working and if an alarm activated wouldn't be able to reach to switch it off. Lots of discussions went between the Switchboard Manager, Rose and the Estates Manager about how to overcome this problem.   They talked about rewiring the system onto a lower board or building a ramp to allow me to wheel up to reach (Would have been a steep ramp as space was restricted) Now to me, having lived through the years of discrimination etc I'm thinking this is way too much trouble for one part time employee. Of course I didn't really appreciate the legal repercussions from the DDA if the hospital first offered me the job then changed their minds because of a 6ft alarm board. As it happens, I came up with my own solution. A wooden stick with a rubber thimblette stuck on the end (like they use for counting money) Simple, cheap and it worked. The only thing I did need help with was the black board where every day the on call doctors were listed but as I never worked an early shift on my own there was always someone else to perform that daily task.

I felt almost guilty when after just 18 months in that role I left to join Leicestershire Police.

The Purple Pound

The 'Purple Pound' is a term used to describe the spending power of disabled people and their families and according to statistics provided by the Extra Costs Commission three quarters of disabled people have left a shop or business because of poor customer service or lack of disability awareness. Statistics have shown that it costs disabled people £550 more a month than their able bodied counterparts.

So I started thinking, what do I spend my £550 a month on that my imaginary able bodied friend, let's call him "Eric" wouldn't? I expect its partly because I don't have the same choices and whereas Eric can pop into the local charity shop or market and pick up a bargain, I may not be able to, maybe this is because there are steps involved, or the lack of space once inside, or there isn't any suitable parking. I tend to stick to the dead certs if I'm shopping. I know that Fosse Park in Leicester has free disabled parking, automatic doors on their shop entrances and it's all on one level, no potholes or kerbs that think they are dropped but probably aren't. But the choice of shops is limited.

I don't go into Leicester town centre anymore because my wheelchair adapted vehicle won't fit under the barriers in the multi storey car parks that Leicester City provides. Consequently not being able to park means I don't visit the Market either. My vehicle is quite high because I needed an electric tail lift. I don't have an electric chair that would assist me getting up a ramp in a smaller car, such as a Citroen Berlingo which is a popular choice for disabled people. Therefore my choice of vehicle was limited. Ah but I could go further afield than Leicester and find a market that does have suitable parking….. But wait doesn't that mean I'm spending more on fuel than Eric?

Clothes shopping; some shops don't have accessible changing rooms for me to try the garment on. I take it home, try it on and it doesn't fit so I take it back. More fuel money.

Shoes; I can't wear shoes from a shoe shop. I can only buy them from a specialist company due to the shape of my feet. A pair of slippers starts at £37 a pair so that gives an idea of the cost of a pair of shoes.

What about heating bills? I imagine that I feel the cold more than Eric does. Poor circulation and the lack of movement generally do mean that I probably have my heating on more often and higher than Eric does.

Hotels and holidays in general may also contribute towards my £550

Eric can go to booking.com and find the cheapest accommodation for the place and dates that he wishes to travel to. Not so me. Yes I can put a filter on my search to only show Wheelchair Accessible accommodation but this narrows my search down from 100's of options to 10 maybe. I'm not moaning about this, obviously I have been in this position all my life. I understand that not every building could possibly ever provide 100% integration. Listed buildings for example, it's just not possible to alter the facade to insert a ramp outside a beautifully crafted 100 year old stone steps. I agree that a concrete ramp with chrome handrails is not nearly as pleasing to look at. However, what I do object to is this. Eric puts in his search that he wants to go to Norwich for a one night stay. Up pop 76 options for his chosen date.

Cheapest being £25. I make the same search select the filter option for Wheelchair accessible accommodation. Up pop seven options for my chosen date. Cheapest being £85. Then having found my seven options I check out available rooms at those seven options. Can I tell what the wheelchair accessible facilities are? Yes. Can I tell if they have one of those rooms for the date I want? No. I have to ring them …. Again more expense for me that Eric doesn't have. In fact I only know of two hotel chains that will let me reserve a wheelchair accessible room directly from their websites, Premier Inn and Travelodge will let me select from a drop down menu "Accessible" and then complete my reservation without having to make any calls. So if they can do it, why can't they all?

Ok so there are perks, it's not all doom and gloom. We have the "Carers go for free if accompanying a disabled person" situation. The "Free parking for Blue Badge Holders" in some car parks. Many attractions will give concessions for disabled persons if their facilities are not 100% accessible. Stately homes are a good example of this. I can't get round the whole building so I don't pay as much - fair enough.

Eating out, another example of less choice and choosing the safe options. I sometimes get told by a friend or colleague that they've been to a lovely little bistro were the food was amazing and the ambience awesome. "Is it accessible" I ask - "Oh, I didn't really notice" or "There was a couple of steps, but I'm sure they would be able to get you in" or "Yes, there weren't any steps but the toilet was down a flight of stairs" are some of the answers. I once had a boss who booked a restaurant for our Christmas party. I asked if it was accessible and he told me that the room he had booked was upstairs but that the owner was a friend of his so it would be no trouble to carry me up there.

So with this in mind, I tend to play it safe and assume that if it's a bigger branded place it will be OK and have accessible toilets. Bigger brand names tend to cost more too. It's not that I want to be difficult. I hate the fuss and embarrassment of going somewhere and not being able to get in. Also the room inside the smaller places can make it awkward to get to a table. There is nothing worse than interrupting people in the middle of their meal and asking them to move so that I can get through to my table. Some people are just rude. Once in a pub for a meal with friends there wasn't a lot of room to get past due to the layout of the tables. "If your wheelchair wasn't in the way people could get by" was the comment. Oh so I'm sorry I should have left it in the car and crawled in perhaps. Now obviously that isn't what I said but it would have given him something to think about.

If I book a table online, I will put in the notes where it asks for special requirements that one of our party is a wheelchair user and could they bear this in mind when reserving the table. Sometimes they do and sometimes they don't. Cafe Rouge at Covent Garden was one where they overlooked my request so on arrival they looked a little surprised. However, to compensate, in their eyes, they gave me and my party a double table at the back of the room where we couldn't be in the way!!

I tried to book a last minute mini cruise. P & O had a really good deal on for a three nighters to Bruges. It was only a few weeks away so I rang P & O and asked if they had an accessible cabin. Yes I was told. But when she gave me the price it wasn't the bargain that was being advertised. I asked why and she said that the bargain was only for specific grades off cabin and that they didn't have wheelchair accessible cabins of that grade. Yes I complained and was informed that it was a "training issue". Now how many times has that been used as an excuse I wonder?

Another time I have found I must pay more is at our local car boot. Booters arriving in cars are charged £7 but because my vehicle is so big they charge £10 treating is as a van. We have no more stuff to sell than you can pack into a car so it seems a little unfair but we still pay and just get on with it.

So £550 a month for me? Maybe not every month but if Eric and I compared notes over a year I expect he would be spending a hell of lot less than me.

Wedded Non-bliss

1980-1983

When I was growing up I remember people saying that everyone can remember where they were and what they were doing when they heard the news that J F Kennedy, 35th President of the United States, had been assassinated in 1963. Well, I remember where I was and what I was doing when I heard that John Lennon had been murdered. Shot on the steps of the Dakota Building in New York by Mark Chapman. Many people likened the outpouring of grief and devastation to the shooting of President Kennedy. I heard the news of John Lennon's death from Radio 1 in my bedroom. I went straight into town to buy his latest LP. Of course it went straight to number 1 in the charts.

Anyway, this was also the day I met the man who was to become my first husband. Eamon. I had been to an 18th birthday party with a friend and we left early to go for chips. The chippy was called "Seaview" Fish and Chip Shop. Oddly you can't see the sea from Narborough Road in Leicester; it's about 100 miles away. Tina went in to get the chips and I waited in the car. I could see her chatting to two men inside. The men came out and one of them leaned into the car and said "You're nice" Yes I know, hardly endearing but it was enough. He had blue eyes and I love blue eyes in a man. My dad had piercing blue eyes and me and mum loved Frank Sinatra, another blue eyed man. We chatted about Worzel Gummidge and he bought me a Worzel Gummidge doll for Christmas a few weeks later.

I liked having a steady boyfriend. It made me feel "normal" He told me he was a self employed Panel Beater and had a workshop in Burton on The Wolds. He lived in Syston with his mum and two younger brothers while his elder 2 brothers lived in Northern Ireland. His dad had been killed in an industrial accident in a factory in Coventry. Whilst cleaning inside an industrial dryer someone mistakenly switched it on. Eamon didn't like to talk about it. He was charming, and he made a good impression on my parents. He had a past, of course. He told me he went to live in Amsterdam to dry out following a spell as an alcoholic. Ok so now I know that you can't temporarily be an alcoholic and then simply stop but when you're in love you only see what you want to see.

I don't remember an actual proposal it just seemed that after a few months we were buying a house and planning a wedding. Our home was a small new build bungalow on a housing estate in Rushey Mead. Leicester. All the roads were named after professional golfers and ours was Marsh Close. The wedding was planned for 9th January 1982. In July 1981 I watched the wedding of Prince Charles and Diana Spencer and dreamed of my day. My wedding dress was brought from a lovely little bridal boutique on Market Street in Leicester called Leah Marks. I think my mum paid for it. It was the days when the tradition of the Bride's parents paying for everything was still very much the case. They also chose the venue for the reception, the menus and the guest list. I had four bridesmaids. My best friend from Treloars, Sally, my cousin Diana from Norwich, my 10yr old cousin Helen and parents friends daughter Georgina who was three. I don't think I had an awful lot of say but as they were paying I let them take charge. He, on the other hand said he would take responsibility for the car, the best man, ushers and the honeymoon. These tasks, traditionally, being the responsibility of the groom.

Oh my word, my parents faces when they saw the best man and the chauffeur. Eamon had a friend who had access to a Rolls Royce (don't ask) He didn't, however have access to a suit and as this was the full top hat and tails affair you can imagine how it went down when he turned up in a bottle green jacket, knitted tank top, and ripped trousers. Nice car though. The best man didn't fare much better. Admittedly his attire fitted the bill as he was in the hired top hat and tails. When I met him I thought oh so this is the guy that Worzel Gummidge was modelled on.

Seems harsh and small minded now that I am criticizing appearance but these were different times.

Parents had invested a lot of time and money into the planning and cost of the wedding of their only daughter and I kept hearing them say "well you only do it once" *ahem*. And so parents and I were more concerned about how these guys would look in the official photographs that would be preserved forever in my life when we lived happily ever after. Still nothing we could do about it as on the day we had a much bigger problem to deal with. No amount of money or planning can make any difference if Big G, the man above, decides we will have snow. Not just a flutter but days and days of the stuff. Some guests didn't even make it. Now, snow is bad to drive in. It's hard to walk in too. But with crutches and a long white dress it's almost a non starter. My vision of walking through the church gate, along the path up to the door and making a gracious, elegant entrance to the sound Wagner's here comes the bride were somewhat thwarted. I didn't fall but it wasn't easy. My dad had given me Vodka back at the house after everyone left for the church. He said, drink this it's the only thing they won't smell on your breath! Now, if he had said to me" you don't have to go through with this if you don't want to" I might have grabbed the bottle downed the vodka and told him. "No I don't want to go through with it" The snow was a sign!

You see, by January 1982 I had discovered that true alcoholics can't be cured. They can be managed and treated with assistance but never actually cured. I desperately wanted to change my mind but it was too late. Parents had put so much in. Not just money but they were so proud that I was getting married and continuing my journey to live a normal life despite the disability. The expectation would be that I would marry and provide them with grandchildren and we would all live happily ever after. How could I let them down?

Eamon had given up his business and had taken a job as an insurance salesman canvassing door to door selling savings policies to people who didn't want or need them. It was commission only but if he did make a sale it was good money. And whatever else, he was a good salesman. He charmed the customers the same way he charmed me and my parents. I was working as an insurance clerk. Mine was the only regular money and barely covered the mortgage on our bungalow. We managed though but it wasn't the lifestyle I had been brought into. I had been spoilt. Taking washing to a launderette was ok at first. It wasn't the snobbery or the fact we didn't have a washing machine that was the issue. It was the practicalities of it. Washing is heavy. I would drive to the launderette and park as near as possible but then have to make several journeys back and forth to get it inside. My cousin Helen (bridesmaid) would come with me sometimes. He didn't help, I could never find him.

I tried, really I did. But when the only money left over is spent on whisky it's hard.

I remember Helen's mum, my aunt, saying to mum that I didn't look happy for someone who had just got married.

Then Eamon decided to go self employed again. He wanted to start his own insurance business. This was a fabulous idea or so I thought at the time. He asked my dad to invest and charmed him into believing it couldn't possibly fail. Melrose Investments was born. He rented (with my dad's money) a lovely little office on New Walk in Leicester.

New Walk was originally built in 1785 as a pedestrian promenade with houses first appearing in the 1800's to late Victorian times. This almost a mile long stretch was tree lined with small green areas, popular with nannies, and iron railings around each property. It was once described by a resident as "The only solely respectable street in Leicester" The houses were designed for large families with servants but by the 1970's most of these houses had been converted into commercial properties filled with the likes of solicitors, accountants and other such professionals. My dad in fact had an office in one of these properties in the mid to late 1970's when he first became self employed. We had a ground floor room and a kitchen and bathroom. Oh I felt like I was definitely on my way to making millions! A desk, telephone and a whiteboard. That was all we needed to build our empire. Everything was going to be ok. Melrose Investments was going to make me financially comfortable again and back to where I belonged. First thing on my shopping list was a washing machine.

The way it worked was we advertised in the Leicester Mercury for "Canvassers" with the promise of making them rich. Once recruited, they would be given an "Eamon motivational, charm school" style pep talk. He bought a second hand old 12 seater limousine and Canvassers would be driven out to an estate (usually Council) and left there for several hours before being picked up again. The following day they would return to the office and submit all the application forms they had gained. The potential customer would have 14 days to change their mind which most of them did. To be honest, most "customers" only filled in the form to get the canvasser out or their houses. The canvasser would only be paid if the customer did not cancel and made at least two payments. And when I say "get paid" they rarely did. Most canvassers would leave after the first couple of weeks and therefore forfeit their commission. Dodgy? Yes it was. Fraudulent? Probably! I was 20, so young and far away from the comfort zone of my family and I could overlook the other side to him if he could become successful. If he made a go of this and was a success he would be happy. And if he was happy I would be safe. Then I would be able to believe I had made the right decision.

By 1983 after one year of marriage everything was rapidly going downhill. I had been made redundant from my job and he only had a handful of canvassers. We couldn't pay the mortgage and he couldn't pay the rent on the office. But what does any of that matter when you have Johnny Walker as a best mate? Oh and a wife who has wealthy parents? Except that my pride wouldn't let me admit to them that it was all going wrong. I only ever wanted to prove to them I was a success so they would be proud. So much bluffing and covering up is exhausting. I started as an Avon Rep. Again only commission but I was doing something away from the house. I built a good little business from it that gave me a little pocket money of my own. The bailiffs came to the office on New Walk and seized the desk, whiteboard and kettle in payment for missed rent. Dad's investment went very quickly down the pan.

We hadn't paid the mortgage on the bungalow either for months and were receiving repossession notices from the Leicester Building Society. And where was he? Oh yes with his mate again Johnny Walker. One day, after I refused again to ask parents for more money he forced me into the car and drove me to their house. He said, here she is you can have her back. I assured them I was fine and that we had just had a row. Dad then drove me back home again. He was asleep when I got there so at least the argument was over for that day.

And so, I sort of lived a double life. Convincing parents everything was good and I was happy. At home afraid of what mood he would be in and what would happen next. Actually Johnny Walker turned out to be a kind of friend to me too. He would ensure that Eamon would sleep. Ok so the bit before the sleep wasn't nice, but Eamon sleeping was good. I really wanted to tell someone. I really wanted to go home. But what stopped me was thinking about the cost of the wedding and how much shame I would bring on the family. I didn't know of anyone else in our family who had got divorced.

There was never any blood, just hidden bruises at this point. And cruelty but how can you prove that? Comments and jibes. "Who would want you? You're stuck with me because I'm the only one that would take on someone like you" It's not like we had smart phones. I couldn't record him, and anyway Hate Crime did not exist in 1983. In those days even if I had gone to the Police they wouldn't get involved. "Its domestic, it's between husband and wife, there's nothing we can do" The shame was overwhelming. We lived next door to a Policeman. Gerry, his wife Louise and their three year old son had moved in at the same time as us. I thought they had a perfect life and I was jealous of their lifestyle. I tried to tell them what was going on but it was a waste of time, I knew that.

On 14th September 1983 it was Eamon's birthday. I had been out earlier in the day shopping with my Mum and we went to Burtons where she bought him some clothes as a birthday present. I got home and he wasn't there. I walked down the road to deliver some Avon stuff to a customer and when I returned he was back. I knew straight away. The atmosphere! His face! All the signs were there. Turn around and run away? Not practical really but I tried. I walked back outside again and he followed, sneering incoherently and pressing his face up to mine. "You're stuck with me, no one wants you. I'm the only one who would put up with a spastic wife". I got to the car. It wouldn't start. I later found out that whilst I had been making my Avon delivery he had disconnected the distributor cap so that I wouldn't be able to get away. Louise came out to put something in her dustbin and I shouted "Please help me, he is trying to hurt me" but she just looked and went back into the house. He said, "See they don't want to know you because you are a lying spastic, No one will help you" I think the truth is that people just don't want to get involved. Back in the house he took my crutches and threw them outside the front door. And then he showed me a shotgun. The gun had been kept at his Mother's house and he had mentioned at some time that he had one.

Now this is where it became kind of weird. He rang my mum and said I'm just about to beat your daughter up so you had better come and fetch her. He told her he had a gun. I don't know why he did that. Why not just get on with it. Maybe it was a cry for help but as I've never spoken to him since that day I don't suppose I will ever know and to be honest, it doesn't really matter now. He let me speak to her but I couldn't get any real words out. She knew that as long as she could keep me on the phone, he wasn't doing anything and so she just kept talking to me and I kept saying "mmm" Eventually he took the receiver back and replaced it on the phone. I don't remember much about the actual beating after the first punch. But what I do remember was seeing blood and thinking, finally… now I could tell someone. Now people could see what he was like. What I vividly remember is the gun being pointed at me head and the words he used. "This is a six shot repeater and you have five chances" I knew nothing about guns but I did know what was meant by Russian roulette. He fired the first one and as it clicked he said "you were lucky that time" He fired again, just another click. Suddenly he stopped. He said "I expect they are on their way to save you so you better go and clean yourself up before they get here"

I crawled into the bathroom and sat on the side of the bath. I filled the basin with water but didn't wash. I just didn't want to get rid of the blood. I needed whoever was coming to save me to see it. Even at this point I was worried no one would believe me, but if there was blood then I didn't need to prove anything. I was wearing a white top though and I guessed he would make me change that too as it was covered in my blood. After a minute of just sitting there I heard a loud bang and my Dad shouting "Where is she" I crawled out of the bathroom to see Eamon lying on the floor with my Dad sat astride his chest and my brother sitting on his legs. Chris looked over to me and the horror on his face showed me there was no doubt anyone would not believe me. Chris told me to get out and I remember saying, "I can't, I don't know where my crutches are" "It doesn't matter, just get out" he said. I crawled next door to Gerry and Louise and banged on the door. It was only then that I saw the blue lights down the road at the entrance to the Cul-De-Sac. They took me in and we waited for the Police. Later I was told that the Police had waited down the street to make sure it was safe before they would approach and yet my Dad and brother had managed to drive straight through to my door.

He was arrested and I was taken to A&E at Leicester Royal Infirmary.

In a cubicle waiting to be stitched my Mum walked in and held me. She cried! I guess this was one of those exceptional circumstances where the "no crying policy" could be forgotten. She said "What can I say?" I wanted to say to her "I tried to tell you but your policy made it too difficult" but I didn't. Then CID Officers came and asked me questions about the gun. Did I think it was loaded? Seriously! So you have a gun at your head and someone tells you it's loaded, at what point would you say "I don't believe you"? I told them I knew nothing about guns but that he had told me it was a six shot repeater. I didn't even know what that meant.

They told me that Eamon had been charged and was locked up at Charles Street Police Station. They said he was full of remorse. I'm sure he was. He would be sober by this point. CID officers said we needed to return to the bungalow as they wanted to search for ammunition for the gun and it would be easier to do it with me, rather than have to get a warrant. And so we all went back. I packed a bag while they searched. I took off the blood stained top and Mum laid it on the floor just inside the living room so that it would be the first thing he would see if and when he was released. I went home with them and the following day my solicitor, David Inman, (no doubt assisted by Mary) got an emergency injunction preventing him from coming within a five mile radius of me or from contacting me in any way.

I saw the statement he made after arrest. He said he didn't hit me; my injuries were from falling over and hitting my head on the fireplace. They asked if I could stand without my crutches and he said no. They said but you've already admitted you took her crutches away so it's not possible she was standing. They asked him to explain about the severe bruising on my legs. They told him that I said he had been kicking me. He said, "No I just moved her out of the way with my feet"!

He pleaded guilty and mum and I sat in the court as his defence lawyer painted a picture of him being a doting husband who loved his wife and only ever wanted a happy marriage. Before sentencing a Court Usher called me outside and asked me if in my opinion the marriage was truly over. Yes, without a doubt I told him. Back in the court he was sentenced to nine months for GBH, Possessing a firearm without a licence and threatening to cause an indictable offence with a firearm.

While he was detained on remand, and a few days after that night, I went back to the bungalow and packed up the rest of my stuff. In the car driving back to parents house a song came on the radio by the Kinks. "Sunny Afternoon". Again for copyright reasons I'm not going to be able to say but the lyrics but they tell the tale of a man lamenting that his partner has returned to her parents, leaving his without his vehicle and complaining of alcohol induced domestic violence!

Another husband plus babies

1983-1999

While Eamon spent Christmas 1983 at Her Majesty's Pleasure, our home was repossessed by the Leicester Building Society and I became responsible for all the debts that we had accumulated. This amounted to about £2000 in credit card debt. Mum took me to the Bank to talk to the Manager about what we could do. She said to him

" Look, this is what she gets in benefits and this is what you want her to pay. You're supposed to be an intelligent man who is good at maths!! You can do the sums"

And so my dad made them an offer of £400 to write off the £2000 debt and that was that. I paid him back monthly from my dole money.

Dad also managed to do the impossible when he approached a friend who was Bank Manager of a different Bank. He persuaded his friend to give me a mortgage so that I could buy a flat. Now bearing in mind I was unemployed and had just defaulted on my previous Mortgage that was a hell of a risk. But Mr Tranter of Midland Bank agreed as long as dad would act as guarantor and I bought a 1 bedroom flat on Kings Drive Leicester Forest East for £13,000. And so with my dole money and Disability Benefits I was able to keep up the repayments. I kept my married name instead of reverting back to Pollock as dad said a married woman carried more status that a single one and I should continue to refer to myself as Mrs Neeson.

I was ready to move on with my life but then something happened that I hadn't anticipated. In an attempt to be the normal woman again I started seeing a guy that I met in a pub who was a friend of a friend. It wasn't a relationship, just a casual thing. He was single but had a 3 year old daughter that lived with her mum. I was less than three months out a violent marriage when I realised I was pregnant. The whole time I was with Eamon I never conceived and yet I slept with this guy once and wham. To be sure I took a sample to the pharmacist and he handed me back a piece of yellow paper with a tick next to the printed word Positive.

What was I going to do? I was single and living in a 1 bedroom flat on the dole. I was still trying desperately to make my parents proud of me again after the failed marriage. How was I going to explain this one? I didn't say the words, I just handed mum the piece of paper. Shocked she told me I couldn't have it. She said that it wouldn't look right as my divorce to Eamon wasn't finalised and he could claim that I had cheated on him. Technically she was right I suppose even though the dates wouldn't have added up. I was still married to him. Mum took me to the Doctor and he said he would arrange for a termination. Mum said she felt very sorry for me but that dad had threatened to divorce her if I didn't go through with it. She also said that a disabled woman bringing up a child alone would have Social Services involved and I may have the baby taken off me and placed in care. Now I don't know how much of that was likely to happen but I was 22 years old and knew that I didn't want my parents to divorce because of me or give birth to a baby that would be taken away. I felt like

I didn't have a choice and I agreed to go through with it. I was admitted to Leicester Royal Infirmary just after Christmas 1983. The nurse who booked me in explained the procedure and that it would be done under general aesthetic and I would stay in overnight. Bit quicker and less complicated these days I believe. The nurse asked me if I was sure I wanted to go through with it and as much as I wanted to scream, "No of course I don't. I want a baby and then people will know I'm a normal woman" I kept thinking what if this was my only chance of having a baby. What if God would punish me for this? But then I pictured my mum's face and recalled her words and knew I had no choice. I was wheeled down to theatre and again asked if I was sure. Then just before they administered the anaesthetic they checked again. I wonder how many women at this point speak up and walk out having changed their minds. It wasn't so bad in the end but I was convinced it would have been a boy and I worked out the due date would have been 10th June 1984. It was never spoken of again.

In February 1984 Torvill and Dean performed their Bolero routine at the Winter Olympics in Sarajevo and achieved the previously believed impossible, perfect score

A couple of days later I heard the news that Eamon was being released having served just two and a half months of his nine month sentence. He rang dad and said "I know where she lives now and I'm not finished yet" In fear of what would happen and not wanting to be alone my friend Karen and I decided we would have a party in my flat. We were worried he would make his way over to find me so if we filled it with people I would be safe. We called it the "Eamon coming out of prison party" and invited a few friends from the pub. The party was gate crashed by a group that I didn't know very well apart from that they were from the local football club. A few days after the party, I heard that one of them had broken his leg playing football.

I went to a 21st birthday party the following week and broken leg guy was there. His leg was in plaster and he was using a pair of under the arm crutches. Everyone was up dancing and he came over and sat beside me. I hated that feeling of sitting alone when everyone danced or stood at the bar. It was always a bit awkward. Geoff's first words to me were "It's not easy is it" We chatted about this and that and I said that I remembered him being at my party the week before. He said yes he was and was it my birthday? "No" I said "It was my ex husbands coming out of prison party" Yes, that is what I said. Surprisingly it didn't seem to faze him and the courtship began.

Geoff told me that once he was back on his feet again it would be difficult for him to have a steady girlfriend. He said he was so busy with work, football, rugby, cricket etc etc that he would be worried that he wouldn't be able to give me enough attention. He had a nickname amongst his friends "Gentleman Geoff" and it was true. In total contrast to Eamon and his family, Geoff introduced me gradually to his mum and dad and then his sisters. I'd had barely any contact with Eamon's family and it was just so lovely to begin to be part of his life. A bonus was that I knew my parents would approve. A double bonus was that Geoff's parents, John and Mida were keen bridge players, as were mine. Whilst my parents had virtually nothing in common with Eamon's mum, they did have a mutual connection with Geoff's parents.

Geoff was a little worried about how his family would be about him dating a divorcee but that wasn't so much of an issue for his parents. Mida's main concern was whether he was only dating me out of a sense of compassion. She had noticed the crutches!! She worried that Geoff being such a caring person was dating me because he felt a little sorry for me? When he told me I did get upset, I didn't understand why anyone would think that, but he reassured me she was just being a caring mother.

1n 1984 when I was 23 I was admitted to Leicester Royal Infirmary where they immediately operated to remove the plates in my lower legs that had repeatedly caused me issues over the years. After the operation the surgeon came to see me. He told me they had had a real fight to get the right one out as it had been there so long it was embedded well into the bone. He discharged me with advice about going to my doctors in two weeks to have the stitches removed. What he forgot to tell me was not to try standing on it until the bone had recovered. A couple of days later, anxious to get out of the wheelchair and back to crutches I did stand. I had gone to the toilet in the local pub and stood. Then I heard my tibia crack. Oh! I thought, that didn't sound good! I looked down and could see the bone protruding. Never felt a thing and it was just the sound of that CRACK! That let me know something was wrong. I said to Geoff, "I think I've just broken my leg" He took me home and made me a cup of tea, then left as he had promised his mum he would fix an outside light for her that afternoon. Geoff was such a good man that he could never let anyone down. But seriously? Who walks away from their girlfriend when she has just told him she has broken her leg leaving her to make her own way to hospital. Perhaps it should have been a warning to me where I stood (or in this case sat) in the pecking order.

But I had just made so many mistakes so far. First husband in prison, unwanted pregnancy aborted. All I wanted was to redeem myself in my parent's eyes and I thought Geoff was the answer. As it happened I was fine, I went by ambulance to hospital and was admitted with my broken tibia. The bone had become so weakened from having the plates removed after 17 years. After the small blip with the broken leg incident I immediately forgave him when he turned up at the hospital with a wheelchair he had made for Fred (my teddy bear) out of bits of metal and wood. He was tall and handsome, kind with such a gentle and honest way about him that I forgave him and fell in love.

Geoff was an electrician working at a factory in Leicester and he would come and visit me on his lunchtimes once his leg had healed and he could return to work. But weekends were different. He was right about not having much time. Rugby on Saturday afternoons and Football on Sunday mornings in the winter then Cricket on Saturdays and Sundays in the summer. He announced one day that he had always wanted to join the Police. He had served 10 years as an electrician and knew that if he was going to do it, it had to be now. And so he did. It all happened really quickly. The application, the interviews, the uniform fitting and I was so, so proud. As indeed were my parents. Mum and dad attended his passing out parade with me at Ryton Police Training Centre along with Geoff's parents.

I was so happy after having a failed marriage this was all so perfect. I sold my flat and we bought a bungalow in the village of Croft, Leicestershire with a wedding planned for 27th September 1986.

Eight weeks before the wedding I realised I was pregnant. All thoughts about never having a baby after what had happened before were pushed to the back of my mind. I told Geoff and he asked me not to tell his parents until after the wedding. I couldn't wait to tell my mum though. 1 more things to make her proud of me.1 more step to make the disability invisible. People would see me as a wife and mother. Having a baby was the one thing I could do that made me truly equal to other women. And this time I wasn't going to be a single disabled mother but a married woman.

We had a beautiful wedding at the Free Church in Kirby Muxloe. As a divorcee the Church of England wouldn't marry me. And to save money the reception was held in my parent's garden. Evening reception was held at the Estonia Club Fosse Road to which all other friends, relatives and work colleagues were invited. We were on a budget paying for it ourselves as it wasn't really expected that the father of the bride would pay for her second wedding!! The following day we went to Geoff's parents to give them the baby news before we left for our honeymoon in the Cotswolds. "Already? That was quick" was the comment from Geoff's sister Teresa.

Mr Stoyle arranged for me to see a genetic counsellor so that he could advise me as to the possibility of my baby being affected by Spina Bifida. I was meant to do this before getting pregnant but hey ho. They told me my baby had a one in 25 chance of being born Spina Bifida but they wouldn't be able to tell me until 20 weeks. If I decided to terminate at that point it would mean giving birth. They also couldn't really tell me how disabled the baby would be but it would be a detailed scan of the complete spine. The genetic

102

counsellor also told me that research had told them Spina Bifida usually developed in babies conceived in the spring, to working class parents and was usually the firstborn. I was conceived in November to middle class parents and was the second child. There was also a belief that it occurred when expectant mothers ate green potatoes during pregnancy. Cases were high in the USA but low in China. My guess is that these early theories back in 1970's and 80's were based on nutritional deficits. America loving a fast food diet whereas in China they stir fried a lot of food retaining the vitamins. Working class families were perhaps not able to afford healthier options? Conceived in the spring when not so much fresh vegetables and fruit available? Green potatoes? Maybe?

Geoff said we would manage if the baby was Spina Bifida no matter how damaged. As I said at the beginning, mum said that if she had been offered a scan when she was carrying me and been faced with the decision, she may have aborted. What she meant was the experts are saying your baby will be born with Spina Bifida and *may* be severely disabled and *may* not have any real quality of life so it *may* be kinder to abort. Yes I was born Spina Bifida and some may label me severely disabled but no to the other two. I believe that I have had a good quality of life and it would definitely not be kinder to abort in my case. And yet the 80% still do today. Is that because of the attitude of the doctors perhaps? Do they subconsciously steer pregnant mothers towards that course of action?

I decided I needed to know what one in 25 looked like so I ripped up and folded 25 pieces of paper and put them in a bowl. I put a X on one of them and asked Geoff to pick one. Yes, of course he picked the one with the X on. Never, ever tempts fate. So I concluded that it was pretty high. The experts also told me that with any subsequent babies the chances would increase to one in 24, one in 23 etc. I was very superstitious for the 20 weeks. Nothing to do with babies was allowed to enter the house (apart from the mound of baby magazines that I bought. No Google in those days) But on Christmas Day 1986 something happened. I felt a kick. Mum told me that was a really good sign because throughout the whole of her pregnancy with me she never felt me kick once. Mum and I had a thing about a certain phrase that people use when speaking to a pregnant mum. Before the days when gender scans became the norm, people would often ask expectant mothers

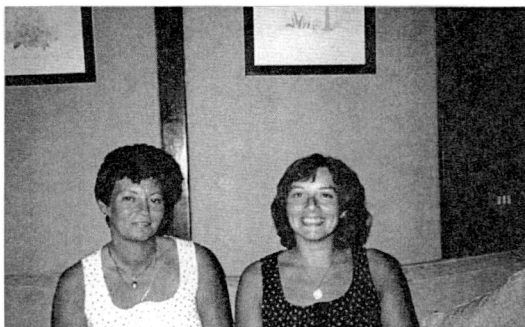

Me and mum, matching dresses!

"What do you want, a boy or a girl?" to which a common response was "I don't mind as long as its healthy" We didn't like that response. Mum said, "So what if it isn't healthy, won't they still love it as much, what will they do with it, abandon it?" She also felt that they were saying that her baby wasn't as good as their baby and I totally agreed with her.

In January I went for the long awaited scan. I met mum at the maternity hospital and they wouldn't let her in to the scan room, I had to go in alone. It seemed to last forever. There was a trainee radiographer in the room and I listened as the process was explained to her and what it was exactly they were looking for. A break in the spine would indicate the presence of a neural tube defect. "Ah, now you see that bit there" she said and I held my breath thinking oh God this is it. "That means we've come to the base of the spine and everything is fine"

We went shopping and dad said afterwards he wished he'd bought shares in Mothercare.

Mum and dad had emigrated to Tenerife by this time so that dad could retire. However, shortly after setting up home there, they began an apartment letting business at Royal Palm, the complex where they lived. This came about because Royal Palm was a newly built holiday complex and as full time residents my parents were approached by other new owners and asked to look after their apartments while the owners were back in the UK. They called the business Oasis Management. They returned to the UK for the birth though and when my baby was overdue by four days Mum took me into Leicester to book some flights so that I could go to Tenerife with the baby for a month in September when it would be four months old. She took me for a drive into the country and drove on bumpy roads to try and hurry the birth. Don't know if it worked but in the early hours of 14th May 1987 I went into labour and she drove me to hospital. Geoff was on nights so dad rang him and he was waiting outside when we got there. After 12 hours of labour anaesthetist Dr May gave me an epidural and an emergency caesarean was performed. My baby was born whilst I was awake. First thing baby did was wee in my face as they lifted it out. It's a boy they said!! Andrew James had made his entrance into the world. I held him in my arms and just couldn't believe that I had made this beautiful, perfect person. I was in a lot of pain from the caesarean though and holding him was difficult. The nurses were encouraging me to breastfeed. I struggled. Mum had warned me, She told me about her problems with mastitis when my brother was born. She warned me off breastfeeding and said she thought it would be easier if I bottle fed. At visiting time the next day mum arrived to see me sitting on the side of the bed holding him, struggling not to cry. She snatched him from me, stormed down the ward to the nurse's station and said "Get me a bottle for this baby now" She was reprimanded by them for carrying him. They said she should have placed him in his goldfish bowl cot and wheeled him. Nevertheless they gave her the bottle of milk. Andrew was fiercely independent. I wanted one of those babies that could only be pacified by their mother. You know, the ones that are unhappy if they are out of sight of mummy, cried, then stopped when mummy came back into sight and cuddled them. I didn't get one of those. I got the one that was indifferent to whoever was holding him, content as long as he was the centre of attention!

One day when Andrew was about two and a half we went to the Co-Op in Broughton Astley, near to where we lived. Andrew wanted me to buy him something, can't remember what it was, but I said no and he had a proper, toddler tantrum. The "stomping of feet, refusing to budge" type of protest. Any other parent would have

106

simply picked him up and carried him to the car. Not possible for me, being on the crutches so I did the only thing I could. I walked away, and began making my way to where the car was parked. After a few seconds he followed me, but when we got to the car a woman who had watched the proceedings approached me and said "People like you shouldn't have children if you can't control them" I was so mortified I couldn't even respond. I was still sobbing when I got home and tried explaining to Geoff what had just happened. What if she was right, I was thinking. What if I shouldn't have had children if I couldn't control a toddler tantrum? After a bit of reassurance I realised that perhaps it was people like her that shouldn't have children. Or maybe she *couldn't* have children and she was jealous. Either way I never had any doubts after that no matter how many toddler tantrums I endured.

In June 1988 a seventh month pregnant lady called Marie Wilks was murdered having broken down on the M50. Her 13 month old baby was in the car. In January 1989 I was due at the hospital for the detailed spine scan for my second baby. Geoff was driving us to the Leicester Royal Infirmary when our car broke down. No mobile phones in those days he had to leave me in the car while he went to find a phone box to ring his dad. I was terrified. I was already completely stressed about the scan that was going to show me if my baby was a 1 in 24. I couldn't get Marie Wilks out of my head while I sat in the car waiting for help with my 20 month baby Andrew. I was terrified and felt so vulnerable. By the time we did get to the hospital we were told we were too late as Princess Anne was visiting that day and they had a tight schedule. Never mind Princess Anne, what about my baby I was thinking. I was cross and upset that no one seemed to understand how much this scan meant to me. The scan was then rescheduled and again all was good. No neural tube defect showed up. Panic over. This time a planned caesarean was booked for May 31st. The anaesthetist told me I would have to have a general anaesthetic as he thought Dr May was wrong to have given me the epidural that allowed me to stay awake for Andrew's birth. He said that with my Spina Bifida condition there was a concern that it may cause permanent damage. And so Jonathon Robert (Jon) was delivered on 31st May 1989. There were no gender scans generally available at this time and so the first I knew about whether I had a baby girl or a baby boy was hearing mum say "he looks just like Andrew" Jonathon was such a good baby. I could put him in his cot and he would just sleep. Jonathon was so totally different in nature to Andrew.

In 1992 with a five year old Andrew and three year old Jonathon my parents gave us an opportunity I thought would be too good to turn down. They offered Geoff and I jobs in Oasis Management at Royal Palm, I could work in the office alongside mum and Geoff, with his electricians experience could be the odd job / handyman. They had bought a second two bedroom apartment which our little family could live in. Whilst we set about looking into renting out our bungalow in Croft, mum and dad were researching English Schools in Tenerife for the boys to attend.

I admit I had reservations about losing independence with Royal Palm, and indeed Tenerife in general, not being the most wheelchair friendly place but to me the advantages far outnumbered the disadvantages. An amazing climate and a fantastic opportunity for the boys to learn Spanish were amongst the reasons to do it. Plus I would be near to my parents again.

Unfortunately Geoff didn't see it the same way. He wasn't a risk taker and wasn't prepared to give up his career as a Police Officer and move 2000 miles away even if it did mean never having to scrape the ice of his windscreen in the morning to get to work. It would also mean never having to work seven night shifts in a row, followed by a quick turnaround to a late shift on the 8th day. I had known for some years that "The Police" came first ever since the day he came home and said "We have a problem with the electrics. We're going to have to sort it out" "What's wrong with our electrics?" I asked. "No not you, we as in the Police Station".

And so reluctantly I turned down their amazing offer and maybe that's when my perfect life slowly began to fade.

I loved being pregnant. I loved the feeling that I was growing a baby and not only that, but I was doing it exactly the same way as every other woman in the world. I could nurture my babies and apart from the scan business I was truly an equal and even though it was hard getting around at times I just felt so proud. And a bonus, I knew I was making my parents proud.

And I decided to do it all again. I say "I" because I'm not convinced Geoff thought it would be such a good idea. After all we had beaten the "25" twice now. Should we be tempting fate with a 1 in 23? Again we went through the scan process. This time it was inconclusive. There was no euphoric feeling of relief when they got to the end. No celebrating by going shopping and giving Mothercare more profit. I had to go back two weeks later and they tried again. The second time all was perfect. I needed to know the sex of this baby though. I asked for a gender scan not because it mattered whether it was a boy or a girl but because I didn't want to be the last to know. I had assumed I would have another general anaesthetic and be asleep when it was delivered. They told me it was a boy and I was happy. Geoff didn't want to know at this point but mum did and she was over the moon. She said boys will always be loyal to you.

When I got to the maternity hospital on the morning of 31st December 1993 I was booked in and waited for the anaesthetist. Imagine my delight and relief. It was Dr May. She said she was confident an epidural would be perfectly safe if I would rather be awake. And Christopher Philip was born weighing a huge 9lb 3 oz. Baby Christopher was like a little blackbird, the nurses said.

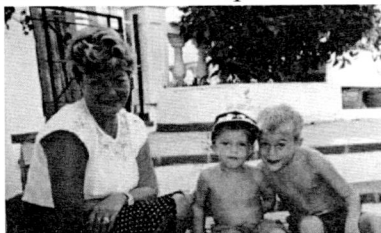

Mum, Christopher and Jonathon at Royal Palm

His mouth opened and closed repeatedly like a chick until he was fed. As my family was now complete they sterilised me during the caesarean. I had been advised that it would only be possible to have three caesareans so it seemed like a sensible thing to do.

After Christopher was born I found it much harder. I developed "infective mastitis", just like mum with her Christopher. Mastitis is caused by a build up of milk and symptoms are a red swollen painful breast that burns. He was about two weeks old and in the middle of one night, Geoff was at work, I woke up in so much pain that I knew I wouldn't be able to pick him up for his feed. I

110

rang Geoff and he came home, fed him and went back to work. The next night, with Geoff again at work I thought I daren't ring him again and so in desperation I rang Geoff's mum in tears. I said "baby needs feeding and I'm in so much pain I can't pick him up". Geoff's Aunty Margaret, who was a retired midwife, came to stay until I got better. She was a godsend. She was the first person to ever hold Geoff when he was born too. A doctor came out to see me and examined me. It was January and his cold hand on my burning breast was such a welcome relief!!

I became heavily involved in the community during the 1990's. At one point I was Chair of the Friends of Croft School, Co-Organiser of the Mother and Toddler Group, Little Crofters. I was on the Board of Governors at Croft Primary School and a Parish Councillor. They say if you want something doing, ask a busy person. I was busy bringing up three boys and all this other stuff. But I suppose everything takes its toll in the end. Geoff and I saw less and less of each other. When he wasn't

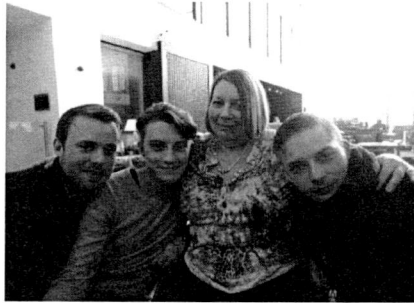

My boys! From left to right, Jonathon, Christopher and Andrew Mother's Day at the Marriot Hotel 2016

at work, he was playing one sport or another. Yes I know that's what he warned me would happen when we first met. I spent a lot of time going backwards and forwards with the boys to Tenerife to my parents. Sometimes he would come over if work allowed. He would take them away once a year when his parents and

111

brother and sisters and their children would all go and stay at a big house in The Lakes or Yorkshire or Wales. I would stay at home on my own. It wasn't really practical for me to go too as the main activity on these holidays was "walking" long, long walks in beautiful locations but hilly and definitely not wheelchair friendly locations. 1994 when Christopher was only about six months old he was considered by the Gaunt family to be too young for their Annual Holiday so I took him to Tenerife and then Geoff put Andrew and Jonathon on a flight to join me for the second week when they got back. They flew as unaccompanied minors and I met them at Tenerife airport. Brave boys! The following year he was still "too young" as he wasn't yet walking. We only had 1 car back then, my Motability car but Geoff needed it to get to wherever that years Gaunt event was being held. On the day, before they set of, I stock piled enough food and drink for me and my baby. You see, it wasn't as if I could just put him in a pram and walk to the shops. Even I couldn't have made it that far. We survived and didn't starve to death.

When I was pregnant with Christopher, Mum and Dad took Andrew and Jonathon to Disneyworld in Florida for a week. When they got back Mum told me about how accessible it all was and so we made a plan to go before my new baby turned two so that we wouldn't need to pay for its flight. Back in those days if your baby was under two it sat on your knee for the duration of flight and although some airlines charged a nominal fee of approx £15 most didn't. In November 1995 1 month before his second birthday Mum, Dad, My brother Chris and his partner Lena, Geoff and I plus Andrew Jonathon and Christopher all flew to Disneyland Florida for two weeks. It was amazing. We stayed in a huge villa. Everything from the beds to the washing machine was huge. I had never been anywhere before that was so inclusive of disability. Not just Disneyland but everything in Orlando from shopping malls to restaurants. Universal Studios, Seaworld, Gatorland. We didn't stop for two whole weeks. There was nothing that I couldn't do as an equal. There was a mail order catalogue in the villa. You know the sort of thing, like an American version of Littlewoods or Grattons. As I browsed through it I was amazed. Some of the models were in wheelchairs. Actual disabled models. Maybe it's not so rare these days but back then it was revolutionary. It made me wonder, why didn't we have this in England, was it because there was a fear of causing offence perhaps?

And then, suddenly one day I realised I hadn't actually got into a car with Geoff for at least 12 months. That's how far apart we had become. Because of his shifts he was rarely available for family functions. That isn't a criticism of Geoff. It's just how it was. He worked seven days on and had four off. We argued about whose responsibility it was to organise a babysitter if I had some meeting or other to go to and he wanted to go out to play darts or whatever it happened to be. I should have been truly happy and in the most part I was. I'd come a long way from the Eamon era but there was just something missing. I didn't want to be a single parent but that was how I felt. Geoff was a really good dad but I was so lonely.

I did something I am not proud of but nevertheless it happened. I wanted attention. I wanted to be seen as a woman and not just the children's mum or Geoff's wife. Even the various committees and other stuff I was involved in didn't seem to be enough for me. And so it was that in 1999 I discovered the Internet and chat rooms. It felt good to have people say nice things to me and to compliment me. I got a real buzz out of it. They couldn't see the wheelchair or the crutches and so I didn't have to explain anything. I became addicted. I couldn't leave it alone. There was a forum called ICQ (I seek you) and you could put in a search for people nearby to chat to. A long way from smart phones with Tinder and similar apps but I suppose it was the beginning of the Social Media phenomenon.

And so it followed that I met through this forum the man who was to become husband number three, Graham.

Crutches V Wheelchair

My mum was worried about me getting lazy so she encouraged crutches against wheelchair at every opportunity. I walked everywhere and the wheelchair was barely ever used from about the age of seven. In fact when I was sent away to boarding school her instructions to the staff were that I wasn't to be given my chair until after tea time. A rule they stuck to mostly during Monday to Friday when the physiotherapists were on duty but then I could go mad at weekends. (Remember I was away from home so she couldn't see me. I was 120 miles away and she couldn't tell through a payphone on my regular Sunday call home) hee hee! Her worry about me getting lazy stemmed from our connection with the Leicester Association for Spina

Bifida and Hydrocephalus. There was a lady member and she was a very big lady. She was born Spina Bifida and mum believed that the reason she was so big was because she permanently used a chair. I remember Mum saying to me that if I used my chair too much I would end up like that lady on many occasions.

And so the crutches still outplayed the chair into adulthood. Even through pregnancies one and two. But by no three I gave in and the chair was used more and more. I had such a stigma about using it though. I thought it made me look more disabled. I would be using it in the house but if someone knocked on the door I would go into my bedroom and park it then walk with the crutches to the door!!! It was as if I believed that people wouldn't notice I was disabled if I used crutches but if I sat in my chair that would be all they could see. The issue was though that the more I used the chair the more I realised how much easier life could be. I could carry stuff. Crutches are great for getting from A to B and being able to use normal toilets etc, but when it comes to the practical stuff they are not so friendly.

I could be quite enterprising though with the crutches. Don't forget Id used them most of my life.

To carry a cup of coffee - place hand as near to edge of hand grab as you dare, hold mug by handle and move slowly!! You won't have a full cup by the time you get to your destination but hey, we can't have everything. Starbucks style mugs don't work!!!

To get my new born baby to the car! Place car as near to door as possible. Put baby into a carrycot (it was the 1980's and we didn't have sophisticated multi use baby stuff) Place carrycot on its wheels to make it into a pram. Use boobs (thank God I am blessed) to push pram to car. Sit in car to lift baby from pram and place in car seat (yes we did have those in 1980's) then leave baby unattended in the car while using boobs to push pram back inside house. The whole process was exhausting but at least is could be done.

Alternative method for getting baby around inside the house! Buy a baby walker, place baby in and prop up head with cushions to stop head flopping. Push baby around using crutch (baby walkers are too low down for boobs)

Carrying shopping could be risky. The heavy shopping tends to make you a bit unbalanced. So often several trips from car to house had to be made otherwise me and shopping would be on the floor. And yes I have been known to fetch aforementioned carrycot on wheels and use the boob method

Then I had an idea. If I got one of those umbrella style baby buggy pushchairs, like the ones that Maclaren designed I might be able to get baby around more easily, they had handles at the sides and I could get in between them to push rather than the straight bar that prams and carrycots on wheels had. The also had front swivel wheels to make manoeuvring easier. Sorted you would have thought.... Except that the ones with swivel wheels all had straight bars across like standard pushchairs and not what I wanted. But at the time my cousin Helen worked for a shop called Children's World in Leicester and she spoke to the maintenance guys and they changed the wheels on the buggy I wanted into swivel for no charge. Then I really was sorted.

The wear and tear on hands was a bit of an issue with the crutches, I did at one point tape bits of sponge to the handles. Which was ok but then in warm or wet weather they become useless so it was easier to just cope without? You may think gloves would be the answer but hey, I'm a girl and I liked rings and nail polish to match my outfits and gloves are ugly. Besides knitted gloves are slippy and you need a good grip with crutches.

Once I started using the chair more frequently I saw huge benefits. I could push a heavy trolley round the shops and carry shopping on the handles at the back of the chair. I could have a clutch bag. I could carry my baby around the house, one handed wheeling is easy if you know what bits of furniture are best for dragging yourself to steer. I was much quicker at getting from A to B. I could have a full mug of coffee, and in fact I could also have a cup and saucer - something the crutches could never allow. I could eat my dinner wherever I wanted to and not just the nearest flat surface to the kitchen. Mum got used to it after a while when she also could see the benefits.

When I became more confident in being seen in public I realised that the good outweighed the bad. I began to wheel up to the school to take and fetch the children instead of having to get the car to go a short distance that was just out of my capabilities for walking with the crutches. Some people I'm aware made an assumption that my condition had worsened. They saw things the way I had, that the wheelchair made me more disabled. Even though I used the chair more, the crutches were always with me, tucked away behind my back. Just in case of any event that needed a more upright me such as using a non wheelchair accessible toilet. Once after having had an operation the crutches were not an option and I was going to my in-laws for a family event. Who knew that their porch doorway was not wide enough to get a wheelchair through?   To get me through the garden gate became a struggle with several family members involved as it had been blocked up for some reason. Something I really hate is fuss and I found the whole experience really embarrassing. This was an occasion when the crutches would have won the debate.

So ideally a combination of both is the best option wherever possible. The crutches win in situations where they earn their keep, but the wheelchair for everything else. Plus the fact that I've fallen over many, many more times with crutches then I've fallen out of my chair - and I've done that a few times too. Crutches don't cope well on snow, ice or wet floors. They also don't get on with wet leaves. My situation now is that the crutches cannot be used again due to leg broken twice and a knee replacement. So its wheelchair all the way for me from now on but my crawling days are long gone.

More hospitals, more operations

When I was 17 my Consultant, the wonderful Mr Tom Stoyle, decided I would be better off if he amputated the big toe on my left foot as it had clawed. When Mr Stoyle stood by my bed post op he said he had decided to take all five toes and then proceeded to recite to me the poem "The Pobble Who Had No Toes" by Edward Lear. He was very proud of himself. I wonder to this day whether he had intended to do that or whether he slipped with the knife!! A couple of years ago I went back to Leicester General Hospital as a day patient to have the small toe on my right foot amputated for the same reason. A young lady nurse informed me she was very new had been charged with looking after me. She said it was her first ward. She looked at my notes and exclaimed "Oh you're having your toe off – imagine never being able to wear flip flops" Imagine her face when she then caught sight of my left foot. Priceless! As the lady in the next bed left to go home later that day she passed by my bed and said "Whenever I think of flip flops I shall think of you" We laughed.

After my son Christopher was born I started doing some work from home for a hosiery factory. The factory was called MELAS (the owner's name, Salem, spelt backwards). It was on a small industrial estate in the nearby village of Narborough and they made tights. A courier would bring me a large box of white gussets that had been made in the factory and the work involved placing a gusset onto a board and stretching it. The board was like an upright ironing board but about half the size and other outworkers would place them onto an ironing board, but that made it too high for me. I improvised and sat on my bed with the board to make it lower down. The gussets were then collected by courier and returned to the factory for the machinists to complete the tights. I stretched hundreds of gussets a week for a pittance of money. I was living in a bungalow and my bedroom was at the front. Imagine how funny that would have looked to people walking by, all they would see was me lifting my arms up and down, over and over again for hours on end! Not that I was aware of that until a friend from across the road, Louise, pointed it out to me!

It was whilst doing continuous stretching of gussets that I noticed some pain in my right shoulder. My GP referred me for an MRI Scan. They considered me a priority so the GP Practice paid for me to be seen privately at the local BUPA hospital. The practice said they didn't covering the cost as I didn't ask for much generally from them.

I didn't like the scan. I went on my own as I did to most hospital appointments. It involved lying very still in a tunnel. I was feeling ok until just before I entered when they gave me a button to hold and told me it was a "panic" button. "Just press it if you feel a bit panicky" they said! Well, if anything was going to panic me it was someone handing me a button to press just in case! I sang nursery thymes to myself to pass the time.

This was followed by a consultation with a Doctor. He said the results of the scan showed some damage around the shoulder joint. He believed this was from years of using crutches. Let's face it; our bodies aren't designed to use our arms as a substitute for legs really.

I was then referred to Glenfield General Hospital. A doctor there said he felt he could resolve the problem if he removed part of the bone around the shoulder joint allowing a better fit.

Ok so this was a different matter. It's one thing to be operated on your legs when you have little sensation, but a completely different matter to work on my upper body. My arms were my method of getting from A to B whether that would be with crutches or wheelchair. I had the operation and then there were some concerns about how I was going to look after my children until I had recovered. The operation would mean I couldn't use that arm for 6 weeks and after that would entail several bouts of physiotherapy. Christopher was at playschool every morning and a friend, Bev, who passed by my house every day with her own children said she was happy to take and return him. Social Services were called by the hospital and before I would be allowed home we had to come to an agreement about having someone come in every day. The home help would arrive at lunchtime, make Christopher's lunch and then leave. The Occupational Therapists at the hospital found me a wheelchair that could be used one handed. The left wheel had an extra hand rim. Using my left arm I could go left by using the inner rim and right by using the outer rim. To go forwards or backwards I used both at the same time. I hated that chair and after the first day got back into my own. I managed to get about by pulling myself along using furniture and door frames with my good arm. There wasn't much paint left on the frames but at least the independence was back.

I still have pain in that shoulder so I don't think it made any difference. It's also slightly lower that the left one and strappy tops are an issue because the right one always slips down.

One of the effects of Spina Bifida can be problems with bladder and bowels. As a youngster I tended to experience a lot of water infections due to my bladder not always emptying properly. When I was 13 it was suggested that I go to see a specialist Professor who was based at The Royal Devon and Exeter Hospital. Well, it got me out of School for a week as I was to stay there while they did tests. How bad could it be? How bad indeed.

Dad took me on the train. We went via New Street Station in Birmingham and I fell on the escalator. I've never attempted an escalator since that day.

I was admitted to a ward and dad left to take the long journey back to Leicester. I was scared, lonely and homesick for the whole of that week. No visitors. I didn't know anyone. The only contact I had outside of that hospital was when I could get hold of the payphone and call home. They filled my bladder up with water and then performed a scan to see if there were any problems. Then every time I needed to wee I had to do it in a bed pan and write my name on it, leaving it in the toilet for the nurses to measure. I remember being physically sick as they performed one test after another. The issue was that if there was going to be a major problem that increased as I got older then we would need to consider me having a urostomy. This is an operation where they insert tubes to divert the urine directly from the kidneys, avoiding the bladder, through a stoma into a bag worn on the outside of the stomach.

The results of that week in Exeter were that it wouldn't be necessary in my case. Instead I was to have a kidney X-Ray every two years to check for any problems,

The kidney X-Ray could be done at Leicester Royal Infirmary and involved an injection of dye into my blood to make the kidneys stand out to be viewed. It was a weird feeling because as the dye flowed through I could feel it making its way through my body like a warm flow. I don't have those injections anymore and I do still get urinary tract infections from time to time but so do many people. It's not a major issue, more an occasional inconvenience.

I wish I had a pound for every doctor who asked me how long I have had Spina Bifida – hang on I'm putting my life in your skilled hands and you don't know what it is! In 2006 I had a Hysterectomy following the discovery of fibroids in my womb. – Now that was a completely different experience. Although the nursing staff were lovely on the whole it was clear that some of them really didn't know what to do with a wheelchair user. Firstly I was visited by one of the surgeon's team who asked me that question, then the anaesthetist who asked that question then the nurse who booked me in who also asked that question. "So how long have you had Spina Bifida?" And to top it all off, when it was time to go to the operating theatre, I was asked to get out of my wheelchair and walk down to the theatre.

Following the hysterectomy there was a further problem with my bladder. From the catheter being removed post surgery to going home it wasn't so bad. But I soon realised there was a problem. I couldn't pee. I sat on the toilet for hours and all that would leave my poor bruised body was a trickle. It went on for days and I relied heavily on Tena Lady for back up. Eventually after a couple of days when at the doctor's surgery having my dressing changed I started to cry. The nurse, thinking she had hurt me quickly apologised. "I can't pee" was all I could manage to say. Within hours I was admitted to Leicester General Hospital Urology Ward where they inserted a catheter and emptied my bladder. I was comfortable for the first time in over a week. I was really scared that this now meant that I would have to have the operation that had been deemed unnecessary all those years ago, the Urostomy. Had my bladder finally let me down? Was it having a chuckle to itself saying "Well you lasted longer than they thought you would girl?"! The Urology specialist nurse came to see me on the ward. She explained why this was happening and that it *almost* definitely wasn't permanent. She told me that having the hysterectomy would mean that the bladder will have been disturbed. She said that the bladder is a very "mardy" (predominantly an East Midlands word meaning sulky or grumpy) organ and doesn't like being messed with. Ok so what can we do to please my sulky bladder and get it working with me again? The lovely nurse said I would need to re train it. She described it to me as being like a balloon that had deflated. We need to persuade to stretch again. A normal bladder will hold between 400 to 600mls. Mine was managing a paltry 5mls at most, a mere dribble, and then, thinking it was too full, would leak.

To achieve this retraining it involved being taught how to self catheterise. Insert a small catheter into my urethra and drain the urine into a jug. The jug would then be measured to check how much was coming out. It wasn't easy but once I'd got the hang of it I was allowed home. The alternative was to stay in hospital until my bladder was happy again. Every time I felt the urge to wee I would insert a catheter and measure the amount, record the amount on a chart and wait for the nurse to ring me so that she could monitor what was happening. When I was running out of the catheters I had a number to ring and replacements would be delivered the next day. It took about six weeks but eventually I was back to normal and my bladder and I were friends again. I made a promise to it to try and never to upset it again.

Having virtually no sensation in my lower limbs has caused me many problems. I don't seem to get on well with radiators. Whilst in Leicester Royal Infirmary Maternity Hospital when Jonathon was born I was in a side room with its own bathroom. The red hot radiator was next to the toilet and I hadn't realised that my leg was resting against it. The first I knew was seeing this huge blister below my right knee. It was about 4cms in length. The blister eventually burst but took an age to heal.

Another time, aged about 17 I was sitting on a windowsill above a radiator in my parents lounge and didn't know I had burnt my thigh, just below the buttock, until later when I felt a hole there. Although it's below the knee where I have no sensation at all, I also have limited feeling in my upper legs too. A Dash to A&E was in order where there was talk of plastic surgery as a means of healing. But as it was the upper leg where the circulation was much better than the lower limbs it seemed to heal by itself. Now you would have thought by the time I reached 40 plus I would have learnt about hot radiators. Apparently not so. The bungalow Graham and I were living in, in 2009 had radiator pipes that ran along just above the top of the skirting boards. I was drying my hair one day and didn't know that my big toe, right foot obviously as left one was long gone, was wedged in between the two pipes. Of course the radiator was on. Of course I couldn't feel a thing. First I knew was getting dressed afterwards and seeing two blisters that had appeared. Here we go again! It took months of district nurse dressings for that one to heal. I also have scars from splashed boiling water from kettles that have resulted in blisters but it doesn't really matter. It's not like I feel the need to show them off anytime

The Dropped Kerb Phenomenon

Have you ever experienced the Phantom Step Phenomenon? I obviously haven't but from what I hear, it's pretty scary for about 3 seconds and feels like you've fallen through the floor. Those of us lucky enough to never experience it have our own phenomenon.

I call this the Phantom Dropped Kerb Phenomenon.

That is crossing the road and seeing a single dropped kerb stone. Usually in front of driveways, shop entrances and road crossings. Then, as I confidently wheel towards it, I prepare to grace my presence onto the pavement. Bang. It's like hitting a 40 ft concrete wall.

Most of the times, it's a slight jolt and blasphemous phrase or two. Other times it's a trip to A&E.

I take phantom kerbs very personally. It's malicious. They look flush to the ground and pose as everyday dropped kerbs, a valuable convenience which I don't take for granted. But they are not. They are evil.

The official reason why is unknown. Some say it could be sloppy building work, tectonic plate movements, climate change or devils play. I don't pick sides.

Here is my plea to any of you working for a council responsible for road maintenance. Please, please, please audit, repair and maintain dropped kerbs. If you're feeling super kind, regulate the frequency.

Or at the very least, set up a support group for Phantom Kerb victims.

To you, I say this. If the kerb isn't flush to the ground, it might as well be a flight of stairs.

To those lucky enough to have never experiences the blood loss of being thrown savagely from your chair and trying to break the pavement with your front teeth.

126

Consider   this   my   friendly   warning.

Don't say you weren't warned.

Also, whilst out and about with family and friends how many times have I had to travel further down the road to cross than them? Simply because the dropped kerbs don't match!

Some local council seem to think that they have provided a dropped kerb if they have made it slightly lower than the pavement. This is definitely not the case. Dropped kerbs should be level with the road. 1" difference might as well be a flight of steps. Wheelchairs, in particular the non-electric type, will tip over if not lifted back to negotiate the step.

Oh and don't get me started on those horrible bumpy things. Hate them. I know they are there to help blind and partially sighted and I appreciate their necessity and importance, but to a wheelchair user they are positively evil. My feet won't stay on the footplate due to the bump bump bump thing. Nightmare

Crotch Height Perspective earns its badge

When the crotch height perspective really does come into its own

I bought husband Graham tickets to the Rocky Horror Show for his birthday. He's always wanted to go. I knew a little about it and there is a lot of audience participation involved. Such as putting a newspaper over your head when it was raining in one scene and dancing to the Time Warp. What I wasn't quite so prepared for was the cult following of Rocky Horror Fans and how serious the dress code was.

If you are not familiar with the story, it revolves around a sweet couple whose car breaks down and they end up asking for help from a "Sweet Transvestite from Transsexual Transylvania" Ok so the clues are there.

We had a designated disabled parking space and parked up but before we had time to switch the headlights off there was a moment when we realised what a HUGE part dressing up was for RHS fans. Men were walking cross in front of the car, spotlighted by the headlamps wearing Jackets, shirts and ties on the top half and Suspenders, fishnets and stilettos on the bottom half. We just turned to each other and giggled!! "WTF are we doing here" We walked across to the entrance and as usual we stayed outside so that Graham could have a smoke. Picture this….. Men in aforesaid attire V Me at crotch height. Not knowing quite where I should be looking. Was it rude to stare? Was it rude to ignore? I mean can you really go out in public dressed like that and not expect to get some attention but do you really expect it to come from a woman at crotch height. I swear Graham did it on purpose.

The next time we went to the RHS it was in Birmingham and we really went to town on the costumes. We spent months of preparation collecting costume paraphernalia. Graham gave those guys from De Montfort Hall in Leicester a run for their money. I'm talking the full "Sweet Transvestite" works. Dr Frank 'N' Furter eat your heart out. Me? I went for a much more demure "Columbia" with gold hat and sequins. Graham's mission was to find another female

128

wheelchair user so that he could treat her to the full "Crotch Height Perspective"

When you are always at crotch height you can get a very stiff neck from trying not to look at what's unavoidably in front of you, especially when I'm travelling around London on the DLR or Tube. In busy streets or places I am constantly being walked into. People have busy lives but mobile phones have probably increased this. They are distracted but Jonathon thinks it's because I'm not at eye level so can be easily overlooked. ATM's can be an issue particularly if the sun is shining. Yes they are low down enough but you need to be able to look down onto the screen to see the writing. I recently needed to get some cash from an ATM at our local CO-OP. Couldn't see which options to press so sat and waited watching people coming and going, looking for the person I thought would be the most trustworthy. I settled for a lady who looked like she was wearing a carer's uniform!!! Had to be someone I could trust as she was literally going to have to stand by me and read the screen to me. She was very good, she turned her head away at the appropriate moments and so far my account hasn't been compromised so I'm guessing she didn't cheat.

This reminded me of when I was working for Leicestershire Police I volunteered to take part in a video that was being made to be shown to children in schools around Stranger Danger. This was 2010 The idea was that a child was on her way home and got her bag stuck on a fence as she tried to climb over to take a short cut through the park. As the girl was stuck she watched people go past and had to decide who would be the safest person to ask. I can't remember now what her choices were but I was the "woman in the Wheelchair" and all I had to do was wheel past her. It was suggested that I should be talking on a mobile phone at the time. What could possibly go wrong? I took Graham with me and he said to the film crew that he would ring me on my mobile to make it look authentic. Easy and straightforward! Except that as I'm wheeling along and my mobile phone rings, I answer it "Hello" to which a familiar voice said "What colour knickers are you wearing" Very funny or so Graham, cameraman and producer thought. Anyway the point they were trying to get across was that even though I was a "Woman in a Wheelchair" I could still be helpful to the girl as I had a mobile phone and telephoned someone to come and help her.

Chip and Pin, very often shop staff don't realise or even know how to take the card reader from its holster to make it usable. If I cannot read what's on the screen and put in my PIN number what do they expect me to do? Give them my card and pin number, a complete stranger, and let them do it for me??? Not even if they were in carer's uniform would I do that. Primark are pretty good as they have designated tills and if a disabled person approaches the Queue the staff will spot them and invite them to use the designated till without queuing. Sadly Primark fail with their baskets. Those net bag things just don't work for a wheelchair user. You need something you can balance on your knee and fill. I always make sure I have a shoulder bag on me when shopping alone and I place the bag part in the basket with the shoulder strap still across me so it anchors it to my lap. Works great until the basket is full and my bag is now buried in the basket covered by my shopping. Helpful shop assistant reaches down from their till and grabs basket of my lap taking my neck with it. Argos on the other hand…. They used to have low down terminals so that wheelchair user could access the catalogues and screens, select their purchase and write on the paper before proceeding to the payment tills. Everything was within easy reach. A couple of years ago Graham and I went to our local Argos and found that they had removed these accessible terminals. When we queried this with the manager he informed that it was on instructions from Head Office. Presumably everyone who works at Head Office is over 5ft tall.

My "Current" Husband and all his children!!

1999 -2010

By September of 1999 I knew something was wrong with me. It was a struggle to get through day to day and the only person apart from the children I wanted to be with was Graham. I couldn't go on like that. Geoff knew what was going on and thought that if I had some time apart from him, I would come to my senses and all would be well again. I agreed to move out and found a small flat in Leicester. Geoff even moved my stuff for me. Graham on the other hand had only recently separated from his wife and was happily living alone in his own flat. We didn't move in together until much later. People have said that I abandoned my children for another man. I need to make this clear at this point. I didn't abandon them; I left them where I truly believed they would be better off. I.e. In their own home with their father. I saw them almost every day, making an early drive over to Croft to take Christopher to School and then often fetching him again at home time. I took them swimming once a week and shopping. I needed them to feel very little had changed for them. Inside I was a wreck but on the outside I desperately tried to make my children feel safe and happy.

I was weighed down by this overwhelming feeling of guilt, not just to the boys but to Geoff too. I felt so desperately sorry for what I was doing to him. He said to me "Who will want me at my age with three children" Who indeed!!

I had a friend, who once said to me, "Steph you have everything that I want. A nice bungalow, children and a man in uniform" When I was going through all this turmoil I confided in her and she said "You only get one chance, so decide what it is you want and go out there and get it" It should have come as no surprise to me when just three weeks after moving out, Jonathon said to me "Mummy, your friend "Kirstie" stayed at our house last night"!

Mum and dad were shocked. Mum said she never thought that this would happen to her grandchildren, that they would become children from a broken home, but some say you should never stay together for the sake of the children as it creates an unhappy atmosphere in the family home.

And so we divorced and Graham was named by Geoff as Co-Respondent. My Solicitor advised me to take the house and half of Geoff's Police pension based on the theory that he was only able to earn the pension because I stayed at home to raise the children. The Solicitor told me I'd "Only get one bite of the apple so make sure it's a good one". My parents advised me to do that too even though they felt desperately sorry for

Geoff. I didn't. I settled for a one of payment of £10,000 and let him keep the house. Had I known he would remarry again so quickly my decision may have been different but at the time it was the guilt that stopped me from thinking straight!

Mum said some time later to a friend, "I love Geoff to bits, but he just doesn't make my daughter happy"

In early February Graham and I moved in together into a flat in Croft. It made things much easier for the boys as they could walk to mine

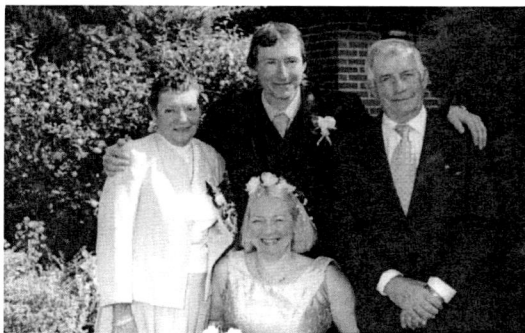

Our wedding! 5th May 2002

whenever they wanted to. Graham has five children! Four boys and a girl and combined with my children they are consecutive ages. Neil was twelve, Andrew eleven, Carl ten, Jonathon nine, Wayne eight and then Christopher and Ross and Kerry (Graham's twins) were six. There is only three days difference between my Christopher and the twins.

When we married in on 5th May 2002 we became a family with eight children. Altogether we had seven boys and one girl. Although none of them every lived full time with us, we did manage to accommodate all of them together some weekends. Quite an achievement for a two bedroom flat. The boys had bunk beds and camp beds and Kerry had a bed made up on the floor of the living room.

Over the next few years we took our big family on holidays. The first one we booked two

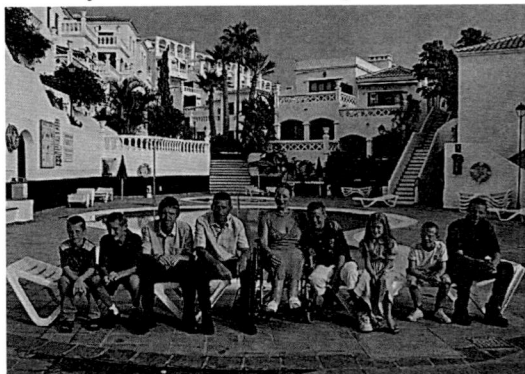

The "Vonn Trapp" family at Royal Palm, Tenerife

caravans at a Haven Resort, Golden Sands in Mablethorpe on the East Coast. The following year we became a little more adventurous and rented a converted barn in France. Then we got really brave and in July 2004 with a little financial help from the bank of mum and dad we took them to Royal Palm, Los Cristianos! That was a fantastic holiday and as we walked down the street, single file heads would turn. One wheelchair with a woman in being pushed by a man, followed by seven children of descending heights (one of Graham's children, Carl didn't come on the holiday). We must have looked like the Von Trap Family from the Sound of Music. I used to joke, "If only we could teach them to sing"

I have always believed in fate. That you may go through life thinking you are making decisions when really it's all mapped out for you. Graham was born on Davenport Road in Evington, and I was born on Downing Drive in Evington. Half a mile away. We were

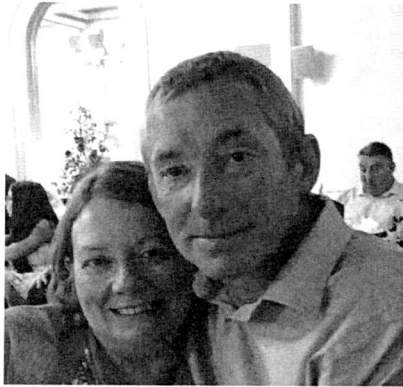
Mr and Mrs Derham

born six months apart (me being the elder so he likes to say he is my toy boy). We would have both been patients at the doctor's surgery on the corner of Welland Vale Road and Spencefield Lane. We would have been seen at the same baby clinic. Our mums may have chatted in the local shops. Our dads might have played darts together in The Dove Pub or the Daniel Lambert Pub. So, the thing is this...... If my parents hadn't moved us to Glenfield before my fifth birthday Graham and I would have been at Primary School together, Whitehall Primary on Whitehall Road in Evington. It took me until I was 39 years old to finally meet Graham but I believe that even though sometimes we take a separate path, we always end up where we are meant to be.

Dad often introduced mum to folk as "This is Jennifer, my "first" wife" the joke being that she was his only wife!!

In the same humour, I often introduce Graham to folk as "This is Graham, my "current" husband!!

Tenerife

2010-2012

In November 2010 I took a career break from work and we moved to Tenerife. Why? You may ask. Well my parents had lived there from 1986 until Mum died in 2004 after a brave ten year battle with cancer. Dad moved back to Leicester but still kept hold of the two apartments they had owned. Dad said if we ever wanted to give living there a go he would happily let us use his studio apartment.

Apartment 5 was on a beautiful complex in the fishing village of Los Cristianos built in the style of an Andalusia village. The patio looked out at another complex of apartments but there was just enough gap to be able to see the sea. Royal Palm had been built in 1985/6 part way up a hill. This was nicknamed "Cardiac Hill" by many who had to climb it after a day at the beach or late night drinking. Mum and dad had been one of the first to own on Royal Palm and shortly after arriving there they began an Apartment Letting business called Oasis Management.

They made a good life there but in 1994 Mum was diagnosed with breast cancer and had a mastectomy. This was all done privately in Santa Cruz, Tenerife's capital city. She made a good recovery and was told that she was clear of the cancer, but had secondary cancer in her pelvic bone in 2000. Again treatment was in Santa Cruz. However in early 2004 she became unwell, firstly thinking she had food poisoning then being told by the Tenerife doctors that they thought she had a ulcer. Just before her 67th birthday she simply said to dad, "I want to go home now". On returning she was admitted to Glenfield General Hospital where it was confirmed that the breast cancer had returned having been underlying for ten years, and had never completely gone away. In November 2004 mum passed away in the oncology ward in at Leicester Royal Infirmary. She had refused to let me or Chris visit after she was admitted so we never had a final conversation with her. By the time we did rebelliously visit she was barely able to focus on us, let alone speak. Again the "No crying policy". Dad had sat by her side for days, afraid to ask the nurses how long she had. I asked for him, and the nurse said "maybe a few days" Chris and his wife Sue, me and Graham all sat with dad on the Wednesday evening when they had moved her from the main ward into a private room. When it got late, dad told us to go home and come back in the morning, allowing him to leave to go home for a change of clothes. As Graham and I returned the following morning, Chris was standing on the small balcony outside mum's room. He turned to Sue, who was sitting by mum's bed and said "Here's Steph" Sue then held mum's hand and said "Steph's here now" And at that moment, my mum slipped away. Chris rang dad and said that he needed to come back to the hospital. I think she knew he wasn't there and just chose that moment to go. The nurse confirmed that theory. She explained that the hearing is always the last thing to shut down and she would have known that dad wasn't the room. My brother sat in that room head in hands crying. I asked Sue to comfort him but he shook his head. Dad was surprisingly strong. No breaking down, well not in front of anyone at least. His sister Audrey rang him and he said to her, no fuss. Fussing won't help me. He was determined that we would all be strong and stick to "the policy" as far as we could manage. The day of mum's funeral it was a dark early December day but just as they brought her out of the church the sun shone, just for a moment or too. Dad just didn't want to live in Tenerife anymore after that but was willing to let us make use of his studio apartment. He said he understood why we wanted to give it a go as he and mum had taken the chance all those years ago back in 1986 and it had been a good choice.

And so on Thursday 25th November 2010 we packed up the car and started our adventure. Yes, we drove to Tenerife. It was 2388 miles door to door and took us six days. Beginning in England then across France, Spain and Portugal followed by a ferry to the Canary Islands and Tenerife. Wisest idea? Still not sure but it has always been a good conversation piece ever since. "Have we ever told you about the time we drove to Tenerife and nearly divorced three times?"

We had booked passage on a Ferry from Portugal to Tenerife on the following Sunday and as there was only one ferry per week it was imperative that we didn't miss it. I had done my research on accessible places to stay along the journey. Not only accessible but ones with parking. I booked one in France, one in Spain and one in Portugal. We had a small party the Sunday before were all the children came to say goodbye. Of course I was sad at leaving them but they were all so independent and grown up. They all had passports so nothing could stop them from visiting, just as I had visited my parents whenever I could when they first emigrated.

Our Toyota Previa was absolutely packed to the roof with everything we wanted to take. I insisted on taking pictures, ornaments, bed linen etc just so that I could make it feel like my home. So much stuff there was barely room for me. At times Graham wished there hadn't been, I'm sure. We left Leicester at 8am in the morning in the pouring rain and drove to Folkestone where we boarded the Eurotunnel to Calais. As we turned the corner to drive on to the ferry I looked around me. I thought what if this is the last time I ever see England. What if we decide to stay in Tenerife and never come back! I was a little sad at the thought but not for long as we had a big adventure ahead of us.

Once in Calais we made our way across France to the first pit stop. It was called "Mr Bed" and booking.com confirmed it had a wheelchair accessible room for us. We arrived too late to check in but we had a code to get into the building. We entered and Graham went to check on the room. Our room was up a flight of stairs with no lift! With no receptionist to speak to we hovered wondering what to do. Then we spotted a phone and rang the out of hour's number. In the foyer appeared a French dishevelled looking man, clearly not happy at being disturbed. I think we may have got him out of bed. Nevertheless he apologised profusely and said that the only ground floor room they had was a smoking accessible room and by way of compensation for this small matter he would like to offer us free breakfast in the morning. Of course this was not a problem to Graham being a smoker anyway, but he wasn't to know that. Even back in 2010 it was difficult to find a room that was both Accessible and allowed smoking. Apparently disabled people don't smoke! We have found in many restaurants before smoking was completely banned where the smoking area would be raised from the main areas by steps. Well anyway, the only thing that made this room accessible was the fact it was on the ground floor and the wheelchair fitted through the doorway. The bathroom was accessed by a step! My washing and toileting needs were met by using the accessible toilet in the foyer.

Next morning all refreshed we set of again. This time we drove to Spain for my next selected hotel. We had our first fall out in San Sebastian. Driving round and round until eventually we got back on track. 500 miles later, and several arguments about getting lost, dark and in the pouring rain we couldn't find the hotel. We tried ringing for directions but they spoke no English and we spoke barely any Spanish, only words dad had taught me over the years so I could order a "vaso de vino de la casa por favor" But being able to order myself a glass of house wine wasn't much use when asking for directions to a hotel. Ok, so we didn't find the hotel but what we did find lying in the gutter was an injured and bleeding elderly man. At first Graham thought it was a bin liner but then as we drove by it seemed to move. He went over and helped this little Spanish man off the road. The man's face was covered in blood and as he pointed to his house and indicated to Graham that his keys were in his coat pocket, he helped the man up and into the house and sat him down, checked nothing serious was wrong and left him. Is Graham qualified to make that judgement? Of course not but we needed to find a hotel and we had a ferry to catch in just two days time. The man was safe in his own home and that was all we could do. I did wonder what happened to him. What if he had died that night and someone had seen us. What if we were the last people to see him alive? I half expected the police to be

140

looking for us by the time we reached Portugal. I could imagine the news report. "British couple, with suspiciously crammed vehicle, last to see elderly Spanish man alive!"

We gave up on the pre-booked hotel and drove until we found another one. Graham went in and asked if they had an accessible room. Yes they did but it was a little odd. Yes there was a lift and the doorway was wide enough but the shower and toilet were in the same room as the bed. Separated by just a glass panel! We didn't care by this point. I asked the receptionist if she would ring the hotel we had booked into to explain we couldn't find them so needed to cancel. We still got charged for being a "no show"

Next day we set off for another 500 miles. By now the sun was shining and the views as we crossed the Pyrenees Mountains were breathtaking. As we reached the border between Spain and Portugal there was a brief moment when we thought there may be a problem. A customs man looked into our jam-packed Toyota and called for his colleagues. About four of them! They all walked around the outside of the van, peering through the windows and studying what we had packed in there. Graham said "oh shit, they are going to make us empty the van" they then began to laugh before waving us through without even checking our passports. They probably were making a joke about "Kitchen Sinks" or something.

Hotel St Julian in Portugal was to be our final stop before boarding the Ferry. It was dark when we arrived and as we checked in I double checked that the room was going to be accessible. "Yes of course" the nice Portuguese receptionist said. "All our rooms are handicap accessible" Well forgive us for being a little sceptical about this but on entering the room we were pleasantly surprised. Ok, so the bathroom wasn't a wet room and there were no added extras such as alarm cords that in England we would expect in a hotel room labelling itself accessible. It didn't matter. I fitted through the doorway into the room and I fitted through the bathroom doorway. There were no steps. And that was all I needed. Graham asked the porter that showed us to the room about where he could smoke and he pointed to the balcony. So Graham was happy too! The following morning when we got up the sun was shining and we believed the worst of the journey was over. We had made it in time. Now all that was left was two nights on the ferry and a short drive from Santa Cruz to Los Cristianos. What could possibly go wrong?

We left the hotel and took the short drive to the Ferry Terminal in Portimao. There we discovered that the time of departure had been changed and wasn't now leaving until the evening. Having several hours to spare we explored a little and had some lunch along a beach promenade. Time to recharge the batteries and become friends again! The past three days, the arguments, 1500 miles of driving and the stress of the tight schedule slowly began to fade into distant memories, with the excitement of what was to come. There was a very physical reminder however, as all that driving had taken its toll on Graham and he developed a swelling on his right testicle, the size of a golf ball. Fortunately it went down after a few days. There was a small child playing alone on the beach whilst the parents were sitting in the bar about 50yds away with friends, drinking and laughing. They were paying little attention to the child. Shocked I said to Graham "Have they not heard of Madeleine McCann?" Madeline was a three year old little girl from Leicestershire who disappeared not far from this very spot only three years before on 3rd of May 2007 whilst on holiday with her parents. Just one week before her 4th birthday.

We finally boarded the ferry and were relieved to find the cabin we had reserved was indeed a wheelchair friendly one. It didn't have the step over the threshold and had a wet room with handrails and shower chair. There was plenty of room but as an inside cabin there were no windows. Ok, so it wasn't exactly a cruise ship stateroom but it was adequate and we could now relax for a couple of days. There was a slight problem when we ran out of Euros. The food was buffet style but wasn't included in the price and they only accepted Euros. They had no card facility and no money exchange or ATM. It had never occurred to us that we would need actual cash in Euros. We asked the staff if there was there any way we could get some and he said that tomorrow we would be docking in Madeira and Graham could get off the boat and go and find an ATM. Well I wasn't happy about this. I was panicking at the thought he would get off and then we would sail off again before he got back. No, no way was he getting off. The Madeira stop was only a couple of hours. We did however have Sterling. We decided our best option was to find a British Couple, befriend them and ask if they would exchange with us some of their Euros for our GBP. We looked around a selected a couple who we had seen when queuing at the port, boarding their motorhome and knew they were English from the number plate. We chatted for a few minutes then explained our situation. They kindly agreed to the swop and we didn't starve for the rest of the journey. Part of the journey was pretty windy and rough and at one point my brakes just weren't strong enough and I ended up rolling back and forth from one side of the cabin to the other much to Graham's amusement.

Finally at 9.30am on Tuesday 30th November 2010. Five nights and 2388 miles later we arrived at Royal Palm.

We gained "Residencia" status which would enable us to register at the Doctors and began to enjoy our year in Tenerife. Now the things we didn't know about the Tenerfians was that married women are often regarded as "Second rate citizens" with the husband being the "Heifer" or chief of the household. Whilst Graham could register himself at the nearest medical clinic they wouldn't let me. I had to take my passport, Residencia certificate and our marriage certificate to a municipal office about 20 km away. As a single woman I could have registered in my own right but as a married woman I lost that right.

We always had it in the back of our minds that if it worked out we would find some sort of employment and stay. If I'm honest, as much as I wanted this to work, a part of me felt that I was always going to be at a disadvantage in Tenerife. I would lose my independence. No Motability car for me or even an adapted car as far as I could tell. I would have to rely on Graham taking me anywhere that wasn't within walking distance. The Previa was high and to get in and out he would take the weight of my legs and I would use my arm strength to lift into the passenger seat. Not easy but it was a small sacrifice for my new life in the sun. There were supermarkets within walking distance but as mentioned earlier this was Cardiac Hill. No way could I just pop to the shops on my own. We didn't have a lot of money, but we got by. Christmas Day 2010 we walked to the beach and it was heaven. Who needs money when you have all this sunshine and warmth? We put the smallest Christmas tree on the patio and had a couple of chicken legs for dinner.

Not long after we arrived there I was approached by someone from the Royal Palm Committee. The AGM was to take place in March and he wanted to put a proposal forward that one of the sets of steps in middle of the complex be changed into a ramp. Now this is something that Dad, when he was a previous President of Royal Palm had wanted to do. There is a large set of steps to the one side leading up from the swimming pool that then takes you to further apartments, the restaurant and a second swimming pool. To the right is a much smaller set of steps that take you to the same places. The idea was put on hold by Dad at the time as it was considered that the ramp would be too steep for a wheelchair. This committee member however was making a point that we are not just talking about wheelchairs but holiday makers with suitcases that may arrive late at night and make a lot of noise banging their cases up the steps to get to their apartment. There was also mention of health and safety for children in pushchairs. So far he wasn't making any progress but then I arrive. I agree with him that if it could be done in such a way that the ramp wasn't too steep and was safe then yes, it's a good idea. The alternative for anyone not able to get up those steps is to walk round the perimeter of the complex along the street to get to the other facilities. I wrote a letter to the committee requesting that this be considered. I was thinking that surely in this day and age of equality and integration it was a reasonable request. A Reasonable adjustment in the name of equality? But I had forgotten that this wasn't England. There were several objections from the Royal Palm owners. One was that people would use it as a skateboarding ramp. Another was from a resident occupant, not a holiday maker, whose apartment was two doors away from the top of the steps. He said he didn't want wheels going up and down outside his door. But apparently banging suitcases was fine? I wasn't at the meeting as I didn't own on Royal Palm but they read my request out in full and one comment was, "well why would someone in a wheelchair come on live on Royal Palm knowing it wasn't fully accessible?" The vote went against my request and that was that. The words "Bigots" and "small minded" were used when the details of the AGM were told to me later that day.

There was an issue with our apartment 5 bathroom door not being wide enough for me but we overcame this with Dad's permission to replace the door with a sliding one and that worked fine. He also let us put in a new shower tray so there wouldn't be so much of a step to negotiate.

People often talk about the "Manana" (tomorrow), attitude of the Spanish. Yes it's true. They also have quirky ideas about paperwork. If you have an appointment at the Social Security Office for example they won't speak to you unless you have every document photocopied in triplicate with the staples in the right place. Staples have to be top left hand corner only, not in the middle of the papers, certainly not on the right hand side and never, ever do you present documents to the Social Security Office with no staples at all. You can wait for hours to be seen but if one tick or apostrophe or staple is incorrect they send you away to make a new

146

appointment. If you want to see what I mean check out a really funny video on YouTube titled "Spanish Red Tape" it's only three and a half minutes long but perfectly demonstrates my point! It is exactly like that. The Santander Bank is where you can go to pay your electric bill but only on a Tuesday or Thursday between 10am and midday. If you're standing in the queue and the clock strikes midday before you get to the cashier, they send you away to come back another day.

Graham managed to find a few handyman style jobs that kept us going for a while but we liked to sit in the bar down the road, Manhattans. Which was a newly opened English bar owned by Julie and Bill Moss who worked alongside their son Dan and daughter Kerry. We liked to people watch from their terrace. Dad came back to Tenerife in January for a couple of months but ended up staying right through until the end of July. Dad loved to sit on the terrace of Manhattans Bar and read the newspaper from start to finish. He never left out a word. Absolutely cover to cover whilst sipping his Fosters Beer. From his years of living and working at Royal Palm he was well known. People would pass by and say "Look there's Bob in his office. Some folk would stop to chat. If Graham and I went for a walk or out shopping we never felt we could just pass by so would stop and join him "just for the one" More often than not that turned into "We best order some food then" followed by staff packing chairs away and then "Goodnight, see you tomorrow" Another day gone spent sitting in a bar, spending money we couldn't really afford. Sometimes, dad would leave earlier than us but Graham always followed him up the hill to make sure he got home safely. To be sure dad didn't spot Graham, and to save dad's pride, Graham would hide around corners and skip behind palm trees so as not to be seen. It was a covert operation that James Bond 007 would have been proud of. Once he saw dad safely enter his apartment Graham would return to me in the bar for a last drink before ensuring I too got home safely! We don't think dad ever knew that he was followed. One particular night things went a little too far. Dad went into the toilet at Manhattens having had rather a lot of red wine, followed by whiskey. The toilets had movement activated sensor and we could see the light from our table on the terrace. After a while the light went out but dad didn't reappear. Oh! "Graham, where's my dad, I think you need to go and check". Graham went into the toilet and found him on the floor. Dad said to him, "I don't know what happened, I can't get up of the floor". Graham, used to helping the less able, (me, and the little Spanish man from the gutter!) picked him up and got him to the terrace and sat him down. Then after a long discussion between ourselves, Dan and Ben who had provided entertainment that night (nephew of the owners) somehow a decision was made. I sacrificed my wheelchair so they could push him home! Thankfully they remembered to come back for me.

You may think I am painting my dad as some sort of drunken old man. He really wasn't. He was a very clever, trustworthy and loyal man. Much admired and respected by so many people. His generosity was out of this world. One of his favourite sayings was "There's no point fighting a battle that it's just not worth winning" He hated confrontation, total opposite to mum who was feisty and would challenge anything she thought was wrong. As a child I asked him, "Do you know everything" because I knew he was so clever. His reply was "Everything except why your mother's so stupid" He didn't mean it of course. He adored my mum.

One night, returning from Manhattans to go to bed I fell getting back into my chair from the toilet. I knew I had banged my knee but didn't realise quite how bad it was until the following day when I tried to get out of bed. It just gave way. My knee was twice the size it should be so I knew I had done something. After a couple of days it went black and developed a blister about 15 x 10 cms. Now had I been in England I would have gone straight to A & E but this was Tenerife. I couldn't speak the language and didn't want to end up in a Spanish hospital. Dad and Graham both persuaded me it was just a knock and would be back to normal soon. It didn't go back to normal. It was painful and swollen for a couple of weeks even though I would put it up on a stool and rest whenever I could. One day when again in a toilet, probably because apart from getting in and out of bed that's the only time I really weight bare, my leg thought "Enough" and gave way. We were in Manhattens again and I was on the floor of the toilet. I rang Graham from my mobile phone but I had locked the door and he couldn't get in. They called an ambulance and managed to get me out. Always in Tenerife it seemed that whenever an ambulance turned up the Policia would arrive too. All blues and twos and full on drama as they carried me out on a stretcher past all the happy, drinking holidaymakers!

They took me to the nearest hospital which was nicknamed "The Green Hospital" (yes it was a green coloured building and not because it was environmentally friendly) but they wouldn't let Graham come in and he had to wait outside with the other 30 people who were not allowed in with their injured or ill companions. He was finally permitted to enter after I had been x-rayed and told I had broken my leg. An Ambulance then took me to Candelaria Hospital near Santa Cruz but again they wouldn't let Graham accompany me. He made his way back to Royal Palm, and I was scared. It was the middle of the night, alone in a hospital where I didn't speak Spanish and ordering a glass of wine as dad had taught me wasn't going to help any more here than it did when trying to get directions to that Spanish hotel. Yes I know we should have learnt some Spanish before we moved but Los Cristianos has such a large British community. As tourists it had never been a problem. We should have realised that as residents it would be different. The waiters in the bars and restaurants always wanted to hear us speak English as it helped them to learn the language. None of the staff at this hospital appeared to speak any English. Eventually an English speaking doctor did came to speak to me and said she didn't think it needed an operation and that I could go home in the morning but would need to go to see the Trauma doctor in Los Cristianos. They put my leg in a splint and several hours later Graham and dad fetched me and we had a real drama getting me and my broken leg into our Toyota Previa. In the end I was unceremoniously dumped into the boot.

We went to see the Trauma doctor at Mahon hospital and used their interpreter service. He looked at my x-rays then looked at me with complete disdain. Through the interpreter he said "Go back to your own country. You need an operation. Spain has no money so why should we treat you." He followed this with "If you don't go back to your own country you will never ever walk again" This would have been funny if he wasn't so rude. I can't walk anyway, I am a permanent wheelchair user and this man who is supposed to be a medical expert is telling me I will never walk again. Apart from that I can't imagine that in England a doctor would ever be brave enough to tell someone to go back to their own country in such a blunt fashion.

I paid privately to get a second opinion from another doctor who seemed to know all about the first doctor and referred to him as a "Horrible Man" This second doctor said it was healing nicely and didn't need any further treatment other than rest and gave me a full length splint telling me to wear it for three months. He didn't even charge me for the X-rays because he said he was so sorry about my experience so far with the horrible doctor.

As it so happens that first doctor was right. It never did heal. I ended up with a total knee replacement. He was also right that I never did walk again! With our without crutches! (he was still horrible though).

"Frydays"

2011-2012

We spent many, many hours on Manhattan's terrace, talking about where our life was going, dreaming about what we could achieve and looking at ways to not go back to England when my career break ended. Initially I had taken a 12 month career break and we were now into the fifth month of it. Seven months left. When I say "we" I mean it was me, Graham and dad. All with one mission in mind, to find a way to stay on this beautiful island without drinking ourselves to death. Dad had a two bedroom apartment that he had up for sale. Once the apartment had sold he said he wanted to have £100,000 that would see him through the rest of his life and anything left over would be shared between my brother and me equally. After a short while on the market the apartment sold.

And so Graham came up with a plan that would mean if successful we would stay on the Island and not go back to England. We saw an empty unit and right near to Royal Palm that would make an ideal fish and chip shop. We would call it "The Last Stop" as in the last stop before you tackle the peak of Cardiac Hill. Dad had sold his apartment and gave both me and my brother a share of the money. We missed out on the empty unit as it went to a couple from Manchester who opened it as a Balti House. The second one we went for was very close to Manhattens. Still within sight of Royal Palm in what was supposed to be a thriving shopping complex but had many empty units. We approached the owners and agreed a price. A few days later we went back in to see them and they had doubled the rent. Unbeknown to us this is common practice. Once you have someone interested go back on the original verbal agreement and say the price has changed.

Now that we had the idea in our heads it became a mission to not be beaten by crooked Spanish businessmen and find the ideal unit. We looked at several but there was always something not quite right. A lot of units are quite small but with a big industrial fryer and a wheelchair to consider we struggled to find something just right. I wanted to actually work so space was important. In Tenerife you can either take on an empty unit and pay rent or buy a "Trespasso" which means you are buying a business that has either closed down or the owners just want to move on. The Trespasso means you get everything in the unit.

Eventually we found what we thought was the ideal unit. The rent was, we thought, doable and Graham managed to source a proper "British Fish and Chip Shop" style fryer.

We did everything by the book. We hired a guy called Dino, who had been recommended to us, to draw up the plans and submit to the Arona Town Council. The Ayuntamiento de Arona. Dino didn't understand about English chip shop fryers and that it would have its own extractor. They made us spend a lot more money putting in a separate external extractor unit. We printed menus and displayed them in all languages. We obtained all the correct paperwork for staff and registered with the Social Security. Adverts were placed in the Canarian Weekly. Further equipment was mainly second hand such as the dishwasher, plancher and potato peeler. Fridges and freezer purchased. Some bits came from a second hand shop and others from the Tenerife Auctions. According to Arona Council rules everything in our kitchen had to be stainless steel.

It had a bar and we had a ramp built so that I could serve behind the bar and reach the till. I think I was, and still probably am, the only wheelchair waitress ever seen in Tenerife. My son Christopher had joined us by this time to work as a waiter. We hired a cook called Julie because she convinced us she had worked in a fish and chip shop before, on the Golf Del Sur in Tenerife. As it happens, little did we know, she couldn't work the fryer as in her previous fish and chip shop they were using a donut fryer to cook the fish! Luckily enough Graham had already worked out how to use our "proper" fryer and had to show Julie how to cook in it. We hired a driver, Darren, to do deliveries and Tracey; Darren's wife was waitressing as was our friend Debbie who I had known for years. Debbie used to work for mum and dad at Oasis Management. We also had Kelly and Jeanette and a barman Kelvin. We had another cook called Phil who worked just two evenings a week to give Julie a couple of nights off. We thought it would be a good idea to have T shirts printed with FRYDAYS as not only did they look professional, they also provided advertisement when staff were coming and going from the restaurant. The T-Shirts were either black or white in a choice of vest style and polo, and printed with FRYDAYS in Algerian Font in an arch on the back.

On Friday 19th July 2011 "Frydays" was ready. Or so we thought! Two things were amiss. The potato

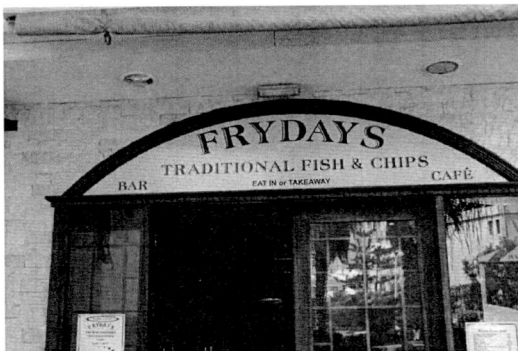
"Frydays "July 2011

peeler didn't work. For some reason the builder had decided we wouldn't need the peeler for opening night and didn't bother to connect it to the electrics. He went home leaving the staff with no other option than to hand peel the spuds all night. They took it in turns, serving in the restaurant for an hour then returning to the kitchen to take over again. Speaking of spuds, we got to two hours before opening when we realised we had been so busy getting everything ready for opening night that we had

154

forgotten to buy the potatoes! Bit of a problem in a chippy really. Everything else had been delivered either by Tenerife Catering or One Stop Bar Supplies and other companies where we were purchasing our stock from. And so asked Darren to go to the supermarket and buy some potatoes. He came back with two 2.5kg bags and said that should just about cover it. Darren was dismissed with a flea in his ear to fetch more.

Opening night was manic. On reflection we perhaps shouldn't have offered a delivery service from day one. I also think other bars had set out to sabotage us. We kept getting calls to deliver to them that night and then they would ring back and complain the order was wrong or the food was rubbish. I don't believe it was. It was the same couple of bars that kept ringing and funnily enough they were side by side in an adjacent street to us. Customers had to wait longer than they should for their food but the reports we got back from that first night were on the whole very positive.

There were a couple of negative comments made on the Tenerife Forum site about the fact that we didn't have a proper kebab meat skewer and were cooking on a plancher so therefore we should not be

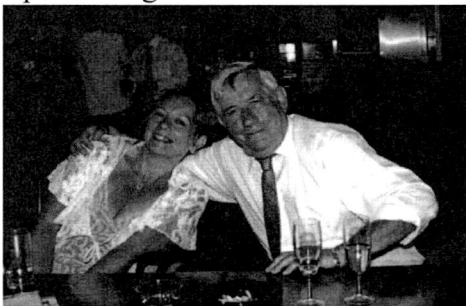

Me and dad

serving kebabs. We weren't worried. Positive reviews far outweighed the negatives. And as they say, "There's no such thing as bad publicity"

Dad would come down every evening and sit and have his Fosters and dinner. Then Darren, or Tom our other driver who covered Darren's nights off, would take him back up the hill to Royal Palm. He left to return to England sometime at the end of July when we had been open a couple of weeks. He said he just wanted to stay long enough to see us open. He told many people that he was extremely proud of us.

We were determined that we would only serve Cod or Haddock. Many restaurants in Tenerife were selling English style fish and chips but using Panga instead of cod. Panga is a Vietnamese river cobbler and nowhere near as good as proper cod. Panga was a cheaper alternative but had a rather mushy texture. Some even sold Iceland frozen Cod Steaks in Batter! We were styling ourselves on being a cross between a chippy and a restaurant. The chips were always cooked fresh to order and we had a serving hatch were customers could read the menu, order their food and watch it being cooked whilst enjoying a drink at the bar while they waited. We even had a cigarette machine!

In theory it should have worked. We were the only place selling proper fish and chips with a chip shop fryer in the area. When we researched the demand, prior to beginning this venture, we only ever had positive feedback. People we knew promised that it was something that the area desperately craved. Someone described how they would love to be able to buy fresh chips, soaked in salt and vinegar, and eat them from the paper whilst walking along the seashore. Staff in local bars assured us they would welcome late night fish chips and kebabs so that they could get late food when they had finished work. We knew we would be busy in the school holidays, as was everywhere, but it was having enough customers at the quieter times that was a concern. We were reassured by many residents that we would be ok as we would have the custom of local ex patriots to support us through those times. After the first couple of weeks it seemed as if many of those potential customers had trouble finding us, or remembering we were there. Only a handful of those ex pats that made those promises ever actually came. It was very disappointing. We soon learnt how local bars could play dirty when it came to a little bit of rivalry. So much for healthy competition!

We had our faithful regular patrons that never let us down. And every now and then there would be a rush on but it wasn't enough. We needed to have a steady influx of patrons. On one night that for whatever reason turned into a busy one Christopher crouched down behind the bar and hid to get his breath back.

One day a young couple came in quite late for a takeaway. I got chatting to the girl and she told me she was on holiday with her boyfriend, her mum and dad and her brother and sister. Whether it was drink talking or not, I'm not sure but she began telling me the tale of how her mum had been having an affair for over 20 years with her dad. Dad was married and had a family of his own with his wife. The children went to a childminder when the wife was at work and the dad would fetch them from the childminder and they began an affair. Over the years the affair continued resulting in three children. One of which was my customer. Wow I thought, imagine bringing up three children by your lover alone, while he plays happy families down the road with his "proper" family. The girl told me how hard it was that she could never see her dad on Christmas day but that once a year he would tell his wife he was going on a golfing trip and secretly take his "other" family on holiday to Los Cristianos.

Well, a few weeks later I was serving a couple and we were chatting while their food was being cooked. The guy says, "I bet you hear all sorts of stories in here don't you" "Oh god yes" says I and proceed to tell him all about the tale the young girl had told me.

I returned to the bar and he followed me.

"It's me" he said. "I'm the father and you have just told my wife everything"

Oh dear! Well in my defence how was I supposed to know?

Why would the man bring his wife to the same resort and restaurant that he would know his "other" family came to? Was it because his other family had recommended it?

I don't think I ruined their lives completely. I will never know!

Another person from the Frydays era who has stayed in my mind is a chap called Deeday. He came in as we were preparing to open for the first time and introduced himself and his wife Beverley. He explained that his name came from the fact that he was born on D-Day 6th June 1944. As his father was on route to register his birth he kept hearing the phrase, D-Day everywhere. He decided that would be the name he would give his son.

Every Friday morning we would change the oil in the fryer ready for the evening. The oil had to be collected by a recycling company. Sometimes they didn't turn up and the oil would go solid. Then they would refuse to take it when they eventually turned up. But that is

Tenerife for you! You can order something for one day and two days later a completely different order turns up. I was, and still am, mystified as to how those companies survived.

If lack of customers was an issue then some of the staff turned out to be double trouble. We made our own beer batter and one night, the cook Phil, was seen collecting Dorada beer from the pump in the bar for the batter and drinking it from the bowl before he got as far as the kitchen. He was later found collapsed in a drunken heap at the back of the restaurant just as customer's walked in and we sent him on his way. Graham then calmly donned the apron and hat and started frying. I spoke to the customers and explained that our chef had an emergency and had to go but that my husband had cooked their meals and it was his first time. One of the customers was from a local successful restaurant and he said "If you want my opinion, sack your chef and let your husband take over from now on, the food was delicious" From that point on Graham was "The Cook" or "Chief Fryer" as I preferred to call him, and we let Julie go too. Darren kept disappearing to go on Airport runs. This is a highly illegal practice in fact as only registered taxis could charge for this service. We sacked him. What use is a delivery driver if he is 20km's away when the food is ready? We let Tracey go too. They weren't too happy. Kelly just quit after the first couple of days, I don't think she liked all that potato peeling on the opening night! Christopher had a school friend called Harvey who wanted to try his hand at Tenerife living. He had trained as a chef in England and because he was too young to get his Residencia without his parent's signature we took him on to work with us cash in hand. It meant Graham and I could take a night off now and again.

We tried everything to make it work. Weekly adverts with various special offers. The Canarian Weekly even ran a couple of promotional pieces for us. We regularly had a PR person outside trying to coax diners in. Sometimes they even handed out free chips! They did leaflet drops around all apartment blocks. We even tried having a singer on once or twice. Customers posted lovely positive reviews on "TripAdvisor" – "Best chippy in Spain" "Excellent food" "Staff friendly and welcoming" "Very family friendly and great food". But without the loyalty of all our so called friends who had made promises, we just couldn't carry on. It was painful. Every time we unlocked the door and walked in it was like a red mist descended upon the pair of us. We fell out with each other nearly every day. Once a month the phone would be cut off and Christopher would have to pop down the road to pay the bill at the nearby Movistar shop. We needed the phone for the deliveries that we were still getting asked for.

Nevertheless I extended my 12 month Career break to 18 months just to give it a bit longer. but by January we were so far behind with the rent the landlord decided he had had enough and threatened court proceedings. He didn't speak English and so he sent the Spanish woman who worked in his furniture shop in the same building every week to ask when was he getting some money. We kept making excuses. It's been too hot for Fish and Chips, or we are just waiting for Christmas to pass. The island is really quiet everywhere at the moment but we know we will pick up. To each of our excuses she would shrug her shoulders, raise her hands and say "Not my problem" A phrase we heard many, many times in

Tenerife. By now we only had Debbie left and she would waitress if we were busy or just clean the kitchen and bar when we weren't. Jeanette had quit and threatened us with legal action because we couldn't afford her final pay. We let Kelvin go because we stopped opening so late and Christopher went to work at a hairdresser as that was his training anyway. Harvey went back to England.

Debbie was incredibly loyal to us and even let us use her wages so that we could buy stock. Graham was doubling as cook and delivery driver and I was waitress, food prep and pot washer. We were a "British Chippy" in Tenerife but as we originally opened during the day occasionally we would have people pop in just for coffee. There was a lady who delivered the post to our neighbouring holiday complex, San Marino. She would park her yellow scooter outside and then one day, she and another postal lady came in and asked for two Cortados. No problem! Ok so I knew that was some sort of coffee but no idea how to make it. As there was only Graham and I there and I couldn't afford to turn away two customers even if it was only a couple of coffees I needed to blag it. In panic I rang Christopher who was asleep in his apartment. Sleepily he talked me through the process. Hot milk, espresso coffee measured to half and half served in a glass! I'm not sure if I got away with it but they didn't tip, and they never came back so my guess is probably not.

One day Graham said "Shall we go home"? I can't tell you how happy that it made me feel. I woke up the next day and thought "YES, were going home!" In order to earn the money to get home we saved every 50 euro note that the customers handed over and put it to one side. Yes, I know in reality that should have paid some of the rent arrears or at least gone towards the staff's unpaid wages but by this point I didn't care. Every day I was checking the ferry prices. We had decided on May to leave the Island just when the English weather would be getting better. On 19th February 2012, Graham's 50th birthday, we closed the doors. Debbie and I spent every day of the next few weeks sitting outside the doors selling everything we could. Teapots, crockery glasses, baskets, candle holders. You name it we sold it. Julie and Bill from Manhattans popped by to see what we had that they could buy for their bar. Julie hugged me and I just said "It's ok, nobody's died"

The next day, 12th March, I got a call from my brother to say my Dad had died.

The day before, I had posted my passport renewal as it was due to run out in May. I needed to get it back or I couldn't go home for the funeral. We rang the Post Office in Los Cristianos and they got it back out of the post box for me. We went to collect it and they just handed it over still in its sealed envelope. No further proof of ID asked for!

We went home for the funeral a couple of days later then returned back to Tenerife to become tourists again. Everywhere we went people would stop and talk about Dad and say how sorry they were. He was a very much loved man. The post mortem showed he had died in bed from a pulmonary embolism (DVT) A few weeks before he had fallen down my brother's stairs and it may be that's when the clot developed. The last time I spoke to dad it was to tell him that we were coming home as soon as   we   had   sorted   everything   out and he said he was happy we had decided to go home. That was just a couple of days before he died.

With all my saved 50 Euros plus a loan from Graham's sister Doreen, we had enough to get back to England. Return Ferry was booked to Portugal but this time I'd only sourced a hotel for the first night. Just across the border from Portugal, in Spain. We could take our time on the return drive as time wasn't so crucial. So long as we were back in time for me to return to work at the beginning of June. With the pressure off we could look around for somewhere to stay. All Graham had to do when we spotted somewhere was to go in and ask about accessibility. We had a budget and just looked around. The second night was also in Spain. A really nice room all carved dark wood and traditional Spanish decor. The restaurant on the other hand was an entirely different experience. Graham ordered a leg of lamb. When it came it had a tag tied to it, like a label. No vegetables or potatoes. Just the leg! I think they saw us Brits coming.

The third night again was in Madrid. This was a more modern hotel and with a better choice of food. Next came a motel in France. Bit shabby but the same price as the nicer hotels we had stopped at in Spain. On the outskirts of Paris so what did we expect.

We went to Disneyland the next day. Well why not? We were already in Paris. Blue badge holders only pay for one ticket and car park was free so it was well within our travelling budget. I love Disneyland because they give you a booklet explaining all the rides with symbols to show "Suitable for wheelchair user" "Will require some standing" "Can remain in Wheelchair" and that sort of thing. It's a Small World has to be my all time favourite. It was my mum's too.

This time though we pre-booked a hotel as we knew we might be late getting away from Disneyland. But we couldn't find it. We drove round and round and then got stopped by Police. The Police woman knocked on the window then thrust her hand in and said "Papers" demandingly. We thought she meant passports but she said "No, papers" Graham realised she meant car documents and handed her our English Log Book and MOT. She clearly couldn't read English so she glanced and handed them back. This was a relief because we knew that when we got back into England we had no MOT and no TAX on the car. Little did we also know at this time that Graham's driving licence had been revoked a couple of years before after some mix up with the DVLA. Not his fault I have to say and we didn't even know about it until we had returned home

When we did eventually find the Hotel I had pre-booked we couldn't get in. The gate was locked and we had to find an alternative. It was about 2am and the night security as the one we found assured us he had an accessible room available. The price was double the amount we had been paying but we had little choice. Tired and hungry we made our way up in the lift to the room. Nice big comfy bed and TV and tea making stuff that you don't always get in European hotels. Complimentary toiletries were provided but they are a bit useless if you can't get into the bathroom because of the step! Again! Now why is it that we have stayed in two hotels in France, one at each end of the star ratings and both decide the bathroom needs a step into it? Could it be a drainage issue perhaps? Maybe they think it looks classy. No idea and so I trek back down to the foyer to use the accessible toilet there. Whilst in the foyer I spot some large fridges displaying all kinds of sandwiches and snacks. There was a notice saying please pay at Reception. I made a selection and approached the Reception Desk where the man who had let us in was chatting on the phone. As I peered over the "Crotch Height" desk, he looked at me, carried on talking and went into another room. I waited a minute then decided he wasn't coming back. Free supper it was then. Oh and the hotel we couldn't get into we were charged for a "No-show" despite my protests that we couldn't stay there because we couldn't get in.

Final stay was at a nice little Campanile just outside Calais. Clean, accessible and cheap. Next day we caught a fast Ferry from Dunkirk and made our way back to "Blighty". Now as I've already mentioned we knew we didn't have Tax or MOT but the law says you can drive to an MOT station with neither as long as you have an appointment. The law doesn't specify how far away from your location the test centre must be. So we booked an appointment in Leicester and drove there from Dover.

It was 12th May 2012 when we once again became full UK citizens.

Would we do it again? Probably not! I have returned for Holidays but I kind of fell out of love with the place. I stopped appreciating the sunshine. When you are almost guaranteed sunshine every day it isn't so special. I will always, always appreciate our NHS. We take it too much for granted. I don't regret going there. Whenever we had been there on holiday I had always said that what I wanted to do was to go there and stay until I'd had enough and then return. And in effect that is exactly what we did.

Do I regret Frydays? Sometimes when I think about the money we lost but then I wouldn't have had the experiences and be able to tell the tale.

The Police Years

2001-2018

If you have got this far through my tales then you may be wondering "Why"? Apart from the success of the Spina Bifida repair operation, why is she doing this? Why am I writing this all down in the hope that others will wish to read and share my story. Well let me explain. In 2018 I found myself with a lot of time on my hands through a series of circumstances.

When you are born with a disability and have the privilege of such strong and dedicated parents you are programmed to think and act as if no such disability exists. I fought hard for most of my life for people to see me as who I am and not be defined by Spina Bifida. I am Steph and I have a disability. I am not "disabled Steph", I am not "the disabled person" and I am not any other labels that may seem appropriate to others. And so for 50 plus years I have thought of Spina Bifida as a bit of an inconvenience. It is something that's in the background. It doesn't need an introduction when meeting people for the first time. It is secondary to who I am. At least that is what I'd always believed until November 2016

I joined Leicestershire Police on 27th September 2001. I began as a Call Taker and after 6 weeks training

I emerged from the classroom and began taking 999 emergency and non emergency calls from the public. The training was fabulous, we were a very diverse bunch and we joked with the trainer, Phil Simpkin, a Police Constable, about how we must have been selected specially to tick the boxes. Black, gay and disabled as well as a lady of mature years. Of course, we were chosen for our merits really regardless of protected characteristics but we liked to tease and it amused us at least!! Alison, Hayley, Graham, Tai, Chris and Marion – we thought we were the bee's knees! The facilities were fabulous and I couldn't have been more content. I had a proper career. I loved my job. Ok so the lift was the slowest in the world. It was only meant to be used for those that struggled with stairs as it was only two floors in the building. The Control room consisted of a mixture of Police Officers and Support Staff like me. We worked in teams with an Inspector, a Sergeant and two Civilian Team Leaders on each team.

After six months I trained as a Radio Dispatcher. Z Victor one to control, and all that for anyone who remembers the TV show Z Cars. Receiving incident logs from the call takers and digesting the information, and dispatching Officers on the ground according to the grading of the incident. Grade one being a potential life or death situation down to a grade four. The shifts were tough at times though. I was full time and we worked over a 24/7 shift pattern. Although the pattern changed many times during my time in the Control Room it always involved working a pattern of earlies, lates and night shifts.

I trained as an Equality Adviser, supporting colleagues with any grievance procedures they may find themselves with. I trained as a tutor too and trained many new recruits. Call takers and Dispatchers. I took an NVQ in Customer Care. I truly did love my job. I just struggled with the shift pattern after a while!

There was an Evachair at the top of the stairs for use in case of an evacuation of the building when the lift would be out of order. Certain members of staff had been trained in the use of the chair but they needed more so I was asked if I would help with the training. I was carried up and down those stairs more times than I care to remember while each staff member did their training. I hated that thing. It felt unsafe and undignified and some may say I was exploited. But I wanted to be helpful and who better to judge if they were going to be successful Evachair people than me. It wouldn't really have been the same if they had used an able bodied person as they could have jumped out if they didn't feel safe. It had to be me as I would know the real fear. One day I was approached by a team leader who pre-warned me there was going to be an evacuation and I would need to use the Evachair. What happens in an evacuation of the building whether it is genuine or a practice is that everyone leaves apart from me and the person doing the Chair, and a third person to hold the doors open. Everyone left and went to stand at the evacuation point which was just across the road from the building. Imagine how mortified I was when I was brought out of the building tipped back in the chair with legs waving around to find everyone give me a cheer. I later discovered that the practice had been specifically planned for a day when I would be on duty. The Superintendent in charge of Contact Management apologised and they then purchased a blanket for my modesty in case of any further evacuations. Funnily enough, the time when it was a genuine emergency it was on a Saturday and two police officers picked me up in my wheelchair and carried me down. Some years later, after having some time off following the operations on my right leg, I attempted to return to work. I couldn't though because it was realised that at that time there wasn't enough Evachair trained staff and that made me a health and safety risk! The solution was to place me in a ground floor office within a different department while they trained up enough staff to fill the required quota. Again I offered to help with the training but this time from the ground floor and nominating another member of staff to be me! Jane Timms was the manager of the control room and as each member of staff was trained she had to get herself in and out of the Evachair to be carried up and down the stairs. I did have to keep reminding her that she couldn't just stand and get herself in and out but at least she appreciated just how scary that chair is. It took four months but eventually I made it back to my proper role upstairs in the control room.

One of the things we had to do yearly was have a hearing test with the Occupational Health Department. This is because constant use of headphones may have a detrimental impact of your hearing. Anyway, the test involves sitting in a special booth with some headphones on and pressing a clicker every time you hear a beep. This would be monitored by the occupational health nurse on a screen which flashed lights and she then mapped the clicks to the lights. Now the thing here was that my wheelchair couldn't fit inside the booth. I stayed in my wheelchair just outside the booth and did the clicky thing when I heard the beeps. What the nurses never realised over the many hearing checks I had in my time with Leicestershire Police is that I cheated. I simply watched the nurse's screen and clicked whenever I saw the light come on. Perfect score every time!!

After six years in 2007 I decided I just couldn't do the nights anymore. I really didn't like them and struggled to sleep during the day. Back then there wasn't so much about "work life balance" and basically my contract said I must work the 24/7 pattern as that was what the role required. The other option would be to go to part time or job share but this would have meant a large pay cut. We were paid an extra 20% shift allowance too if we did the whole pattern plus an enhancement for working at weekends. I changed roles to one that was still in the Control room but involved working between the hours of 7am and 10pm only. The Service Delivery Desk was a slower pace but still incurred a weekend working enhancement. It was a drop in pay as this role was of a lower grade than that of Dispatcher. After a year it was decided that the Service Delivery Desk would merge with the Crime Bureau and I was given a new title. "Crime and Incident Adviser". We moved from the buzz of the Control Room to the building where the Crime Bureau was situated. It was a much quieter pace and calmer atmosphere and on the ground floor.I had worked in there twice before with the Crime Bureau staff. Once when they were installing a new air conditioning system in the Control Room which meant the lift would be out of order and again a couple of years later when the lift was broken and they had to order the parts from somewhere abroad.

By 2010 things changed again when the Crime and Incident Unit was moved back into the Control Room. At this point I took my career break to Tenerife and was away from Police life for 18 months.

In 2015 a new department was set up again and the Crime and Incident Unit was incorporated into the Investigation Management Unit and I began a new role as an Investigator. This was back in the old Crime Bureau building so no more Evachair for me. At a time of police budget cuts by the Government it was always a mystery to me why they spent so much money moving people around and changing job titles over the years. But with no Evachair to contend with this at least meant that for the most part I was an equal to my colleagues and just blended in. Ok, when I say mostly I did have to travel further to the only accessible toilet in the building and couldn't use the one just outside the office door. I didn't mind that so much as it got me out of the office for a couple more minutes than an average toilet break. I had a desk with adjustable height and a parking space with my Car Reg. I was asked which locker I wanted and chose the one nearest the door for ease of access. They put a nail in the side of my locker to use as a coat peg. I never complained about the height of the worktops in the kitchen or not being able to reach the drinking water tap. It was a good thing that the crisps for the tuck shop were placed out of my reach on top of the fridge. I coped with how heavy the door into the locker room was because that's just how it is. No fuss, just come into work and get on with it.

After the Chair of the Disability Support Network resigned from the Police I was asked by the Head of Equality if I would be interested in taking over. I jumped at the chance of another string to my bow and along with another lady took it on as a joint role. We set about raising more awareness of the function of the Network. Its purpose was to offer support and advice to employees' right across the Force if they or anyone in

171

their family was affected by disability. Outside of the Lecture Theatre at Force HQ was a foyer that was used for "meet and greet", buffets and general refreshments whenever an event was held in there. The Estates Department decided one day to change the layout. Small tables and chairs were removed and replaced with bar stools and tall tables. Ok, I don't know whose actual idea it was, but this was totally useless to me, and indeed anyone who would struggle to get onto a bar stool. The matter was raised by Sarah in the Equality Unit with the head of Estates. Sarah pointed out to him how impractical this new layout was. Bearing in mind the public often came to events there, so we weren't asking for special treatment for a few employees. His reply was something along the lines of "It's what people want and we can't have a few disabled people spoiling it for the rest" Sometime later I was on a training course in the Lecture Theatre that included a buffet at lunchtime. The compromise to the issue was that the catering department placed a small table at the end with a selection of food and five minutes before the others I was called out of the room to sit at my small table, with another colleague for company!

The Disability Support Network held an event which I named *"More Awareness, Less Fuss"* I thought it pretty much summed up how disabled employees would like to be treated. Every employee at Police Force HQ was invited and the event was opened by the Chief Constable. As part of the event I thought "wheelchair slalom" would be a great way to demonstrate life at "crotch height" to a standing person! Graham came along too and we constructed it out of long wooden poles placed along the floor in the lecture theatre. The person would have to sit in a wheelchair, borrowed from

172

reception, and negotiate manoeuvring between the poles placed narrowly apart. Some poles were laid across to give the challenge of getting over a small step. Then they had to get through a push door out into the foyer, pour a cup of water (it wasn't really water it was polystyrene balls, much less messy that water) from a jug placed on a tall table and carry the "water" back to the beginning through a pull door. Along the way were chairs with coats and bags hanging off the back that they had to move out of the way to get through, just like in a real office! Hopefully it did help with awareness but what we didn't mention was that one of the wheelchairs had a puncture! I did get some really positive feedback and comments such as "I don't know how you do this every day Steph" and "Wow, who knew it was this hard being disabled" Sarah, my blind colleague did the same with performing activities with a blindfold on. It was good to give an insight into how it is. My work life was fulfilling.

But then everything changed I had a new line manager in 2016. A Police Sergeant. I'd never met him before and to be honest he seemed a little eccentric. He would lie down in the middle of the open plan office and do stretching exercises. He seemed to like being the centre of attention. He had a habit of referring to me as "The disabled one" One day I approached his desk for advice and when I thought he had finished speaking I moved away "Don't roll away when I'm talking to you" were his exact words. I let it go. I'm not that sensitive and I just thought he was ignorant.

Another day he came up behind me and pulled my wheelchair backwards and shoved it across the room. That was a bit too much. Would you do that to a person? No you wouldn't. I spoke to the Inspector in charge of the Department and told him how uncomfortable he was making me feel. I asked if I could be moved to another shift so that I wouldn't have to work with him so much. The Inspector told me that wasn't an option. The Sergeant was spoken to and given words of advice and it was explained to him how he was making me feel. He was asked to stop.

He didn't stop. He thanked me for grassing him up and then took it to another level.

It wasn't just me that was targeted. A colleague who had permission to alter her shift in order to attend Church was asked if she was "One of those happy clappers" A male colleague who was only about 5ft was asked if he had "little man syndrome" Another was teased about her age as she was still working despite being over retirement age. It seemed as if he was working his way through all the protected characteristics. But me, he seemed to like to pick on more than anyone. I would be in tears driving to work wondering what he was going to say or do. Getting home Graham would look at me and ask "Come on, what's the dickhead done today?"

It all came to a head one Sunday morning, 5th February 2017 to be exact. Now as I've said his behaviour could be bizarre but it was selective behaviour. It always happened in the evenings or at weekends when no other managers were around. The office was open plan with the supervisor's desk facing into the room and then rows and rows of desks. He was at his desk at one end and I was at my desk at the other end with my back to him. Unbeknown to me he lay down on the floor and did a full combat style crawl

174

down the length of the office until he got to me. Someone said to me "Look out Steph" and as I looked down he had his head under my wheelchair. I asked him what he was doing. My first thought was that he was looking up my skirt. But no, he said he was trying to find my valves to let my tyres down. I was embarrassed but I didn't want to make a fuss. I could see people looking shocked. It was as if the room froze waiting to see my reaction. I let it go in an attempt to minimize the fuss and attention, not just towards me but to him too. A little later that morning I needed to approach him to seek advice and he grabbed my wheelchair and spun me around pushing me away saying he was busy. A Police Officer Colleague sitting nearby told him "I really don't think you should have done that, it could be considered an assault" The Sergeant shrugged it off. The third thing to happen that day was when I heard him say "I think I'm going to clamp her. She won't be able to leave her desk then" At that point a colleague said to me, "That's enough, you really have to tell someone, he has gone way too far"

As I said, when you fight throughout your life to make people not see the disability this was really tough. How could I or any of my colleagues ignore it when he was repeatedly making fun? Humiliating and embarrassing me at every opportunity. I didn't understand why. This was the 21st Century and we don't behave like that in the workplace or any other place. It brought back memories from being teased at primary school. I felt I had failed. I thought I had done such a good job of people not being seeing me as "The disabled one". But obviously not! It was tough. I wrote an email of complaint again to the Inspector and then made a formal complaint. Obviously being given words of advice has not worked on him and I felt it needed a stronger approach. Several of my colleagues approached the Office Manager the following day to report what they had seen and heard. I felt quite comforted by that. I had the support of others.

A few days later Professional Standards served papers on him for Gross Misconduct and he reported sick.

I felt terrible. They told me he could be dismissed and may even lose his pension. He was due to retire within about 18 months. I felt as if I had ruined his life. If only I had been stronger and been able to laugh off his antics. If only Id not been so sensitive.

I thought that he would hold his hands up and say sorry. I really did. I believed that he would feel bad about what he had put me through and see how upsetting his behaviour was.

I wanted two things. One was for him not to be my line manager anymore and two for him to acknowledge how he had made me feel. Well I got the first one at least. I was told he wouldn't be returning to the department and he would be placed somewhere else after their investigation, assuming he hadn't been dismissed.

The process was explained to me. He was shown my statement and told he had 10 days to respond in writing. After that, there would be a full investigation. Statements from witnesses would be taken and then there would be a Gross Misconduct Hearing where I would need to give evidence rather like a court hearing.

With him out of the way, work life returned to normal. Well almost. You see, this thing was now hanging over me. Ok so I didn't have to see him every day but he was never far from my thoughts. It was the guilt as well as people asking me all the time what was happening. I hadn't realised just how unpopular he was.

I don't think, unless you have experienced it, anyone knows what it's like to believe that you are responsible for another person's downfall. Now logically I knew he was responsible for his actions and not me. But it didn't matter how many people reassured me, I couldn't shake off that feeling of guilt. And so I waited for it all to be over. And waited! The problem was that he had failed to respond either in writing or verbally. I was aware that he had a Police Federation Rep advising him. It was almost like a "No comment" that suspects give under interview.

One day, about a month after making my complaint, in March, I woke up in bed and couldn't move my arms. It was as if they were made of lead. They were really painful to move. After about an hour they loosened up and it was ok. But it kept happening. When your arms are the only fully functioning limbs you have it's pretty scary when they go wrong. I went to the dr's and explained what had happened. She referred me to a Rheumatologist and I was warned this could be the onset of Rheumatoid Arthritis. Great! "Double Disabled"! My Grandma had the condition and I remembered how she struggled with joint pain and swollen claw like hands. Her knuckles were prominent and she knitted all the time because she said it was the only way to lessen the pain. Well obviously I googled it. Don't we all when we're told of a medical condition? Apparently it's likely to be hereditary if anyone on the paternal side has the condition. Yes Grandma was my dad's mum.

I saw the Rheumatologist and had several blood tests done. It was explained to me how the condition would be likely to affect me further down the line and that treatment involved taking cocktails of steroids and injections. It was a daunting prospect. My legs have never worked properly and now my arms were letting me down too.

I was put on light duties at work and was determined not to take any time off sick. I was shocked at the quickness of the onset of this but got through on painkillers and positivity!

The complaint went on and on with no progress. It all became too much. He had a Welfare Officer and a Federation Rep and I had no one. His lack of cooperation made me hate him. Why wouldn't he want this to be over? Was it because he was of sick on full pay and that would all stop if he were to be dismissed? Was this about money? As the months passed by any feelings of guilt or remorse that I had felt vanished. He was playing a game.

Then one day around July time I was spoken to by my line manager. He told me he had been asked to speak to me because I was under performing. It was upsetting but not entirely a surprise. I knew I wasn't coping. By September I asked my GP for help and she insisted I needed to take some time out. I thought she would just give me a prescription.. I didn't want to do that because I knew how hard it would be to return. But deep down I knew I had to do it.

Anxiety and depression are horrible. They take you to a very lonely place. I didn't know it was happening at first; it just crept up on me. It wasn't just the constant tears. Everything set me off, happy or sad. It was more the overwhelming feeling that I wasn't good enough. That nobody liked me. That I could count on one had how many people would attend my funeral if I died. If you convince yourself you're not good enough then how can anyone else know that you are? And the sense of impending doom that something bad was about to happen. In the car, I imagined people crashing into me. If Graham went out of the door I visualised a Police Officer knocking later with bad news. I couldn't read a book or concentrate on a film. Getting dressed and leaving the house became a trial. Graham had to find inventive ways to make me go out even if only to Tesco. I imagined my colleagues at work were talking about me and saying I'd overreacted and I should be able to handle that kind of behaviour from him. In a nutshell I felt like a total wimp.

It was suggested to me by Occupational Health that I may benefit from some counselling. The Force used an outside company. I made the call and was told someone would be allocated to me within 48 hours. I explained that wherever I needed to get to would need to be wheelchair accessible due to me being a permanent wheelchair user. A week later someone called me back. He said that they had found someone who I could see but that she had steps into her house. He said that she was more than happy to bring my wheelchair inside once I had walked in. Nope, not happening! A few days later I received another call to say they were really sorry but they couldn't find a counsellor in Leicester that could accommodate a wheelchair. I finally agreed to go to Nottingham, about a 40 minute drive, to see someone.

In October, eight months after making my complaint, completely out of the blue I received an email telling me that the complaint had been downgraded and that he would be dealt with by way of a Misconduct Meeting, as opposed to a Gross Misconduct Hearing. That was a shock. How had that happened? I had so many questions. The Superintendent in charge of Professional Standards agreed to meet with me to explain his rationale. Basically the Sergeant had mental health problems. They felt that nothing was to be gained by keeping the complaint as a Gross Misconduct. If they had, it would have to be dealt with by an independent panel and would become public knowledge. They wouldn't be able to deal in house. The panel could dismiss him. As Misconduct however, he could be interviewed internally and given a written warning. Not much of a punishment considering he only had about a year to go to retirement by this time. The Superintendant said that they were thinking of me and didn't want to put me through the distress of giving evidence at a hearing and the public becoming aware of what I had been through. What they really meant I believe is that they didn't want the press getting hold of the story. How bad would that look? Leicestershire Police Sergeant bullies and discriminates against disabled member of Police Staff.

It felt as though he had broken me. They had let me down. I no longer trusted them to protect me. The final straw came when I returned to work in February 2018 and was told I needed to take all the unused leave that I had accrued but been unable to use due to my time of. I had just returned after 5 months off sick and they wanted me to take more time to e up the accrued annual leave. I asked if I could take payment and it was refused. I felt completely undervalued. It was like they were saying they didn't really need me. I made a decision. I couldn't go back. I'd been so proud of my career with Leicestershire Police but that was all destroyed, not just by the actions of that Sergeant, but by the organisation that had a duty of care towards me. At my exit interview with the HR Officer Teresa she suggested that I took out a grievance against Leicestershire Police and considered making a case for Constructive Dismissal. By definition in employment law, Constructive Dismissal occurs when an employee resigns as a result of the employer creating a hostile working environment.

After consulting a solicitor I was told that in order to bring a case of Constructive Dismissal against Leicestershire Police I would needed to have done it within "3 months less 1 day" from the date of the discrimination. I was too late. But that would have been impossible due to that Sergeant failing to respond to my complaint for the best part of a year.

And so on the 2nd June 2018 my career with Leicestershire Police ended.

Oh and as for my arms. Well after more blood tests and checks the Rheumatologist concluded that this was not Rheumatoid Arthritis after all and more likely to be Chronic Pain Syndrome brought on by the stress that Leicestershire Police and in particular that Sergeant had caused. In fact he wrote to my GP saying he had seen a huge improvement in my general demeanour since I had retired from work.

Taking one for the team

And so my parents did such an awesome job of raising me to not focus on the disability that every now and again I'm given a reminder.

On holiday in Spain in late 1960's or early 70's aged about nine years we made friends with another family and our parents arranged for us to go horse riding. Dad and the other father, me and the girl all went to the stables where they organised pony treks around the Spanish countryside. We got there and the man looked at me and said "No ella no puede hacerlo" *She cannot do it.* So that was it, no explanation but I'm guessing it was a health and safety sort of thing if they even existed in the 70's. I remember feeling a bit disappointed as Id been horse riding for years but it was ok. Dad said ok we can still watch the ponies. But the dad of the other girl said no, if she can't do it then we won't either. This was an odd feeling, to me that meant that I was responsible for the other girl not being able to ride. But it wasn't my choice, the adults made the decisions and we went back to the resort.

Another time Dad took me into Leicester to the ABC cinema Belgrave gate to see Jaws (I think)

We went into the foyer and the woman in the ticket office said "No, sorry she can't come in as its being shown on screen 3 and that's upstairs. Dad said that's ok she can climb stairs. "No, sorry, we can't let her come in, in-case there's an evacuation. We left and he stopped on the way home and bought me the latest Bay City Rollers LP from a shop on Hinckley Road.

I think he was more upset than me to be honest, but that wasn't the point.

Today I am really cautious about going anywhere I've never been to before. The embarrassment of getting somewhere and being turned away is something you can't possibly imagine, unless you have experienced it.

When I was seventeen I went to see Rod Stewart at Granby Halls in Leicester. It was standing only so the bouncers lifted me up in my chair and put me on a table so I could see. Yes, total contrast but that must be because it's Rock n Roll

A police work colleague was planning a night out at an Indian restaurant he regularly frequented. They had a special offer on, three courses for £15, and he said the food was excellent. Really good value with lovely ambience, friendly staff etc etc. The thing is I knew that this restaurant was upstairs with no lift. So I sent my colleague an email reply to the invite. It was light hearted where I included images of a wheelchair at the bottom of a flight of stairs and a sad looking person!! He spoke to me and asked if I wanted him to change the venue. Ok this is a no win to me. If I say yes, change the venue then I feel bad as the whole point was his recommendation to this particular venue. So my only real option was to say "no, its fine and I can't make it anyway". He said "are you sure and you're not just taking one for the team" Yes, in all fairness he saw right through that one. To be honest it made me sad. I hate anything that reminds me I'm disabled and this undoubtedly did.

These days it's all so much better in theory. Many venues like cinemas, theatres, arenas etc will offer concessionary tickets to events such as "Disabled person and Carer" only pay for one ticket. Saves a lot of money and encourages you to actually go out there and do things safe in the knowledge that the facilities will be good. Im basing this theory on the fact they wouldn't be selling the concessionary tickets if they couldn't accommodate me.

I've always been a massive Celine Dion fan and my sons have been brought up having been forced to listen to her usually when I've been driving them to and fro.

So imagine my excitement when son Jonathon tells me she is playing just one venue, for one day only in Hyde Park, London.

"We have to go, it's not up for discussion" says Christopher

Two days before tickets go on sale I'm reading up everything I can about booking tickets at Hyde Park. They have a wheelchair platform where wheelchair and PA can view the stage easily and ticket prices are at the concessionary price. If there is more than one person in your party then the PA is interchangeable! We needed one wheelchair and one PA ticket plus two more general tickets. As soon as tickets were released Jonathon went on to the general sales online and I rang the wheelchair priority line, whilst looking on line at the same time. Within minutes all the wheelchair sales online had gone but I persevered on the phone waiting to get through. (7p a minute I might add – Purple Pound comes to mind)

Whilst waiting on the phone Jonathon messages me to say he can get general tickets so I'm telling him to go for it. Don't worry about me; I will keep trying to get through for the wheelchair platform tickets.

Jonathon books two tickets online, easy straightforward within minutes. I get through on the phone after 30 minutes to be told all the wheelchair tickets are gone. This has costs me £2.10 so far in phone charges. Ok, so I understand the wheelchair platform is not going to be massive, but why isn't it? Should we not be making more and more areas accessible? I know I'm getting cheaper tickets but if I can't get any because they have sold out within 30 minutes of going on sale then what's the point?

The ticket sales man takes my details and places me on a waiting list saying that I should keep checking back on the website every five to six hours every day in case the promoters release more tickets. Why? If spaces on the wheelchair viewing platform are limited, why hold tickets back? Why make life more difficult to the wheelchair person?

Why should I check back every five to six hours, why are they dangling a carrot on a stick to keep my hopes up that I might be able to get a ticket? We all know there is only a certain amount of wheelchair space on a platform. So why not just fill it up and get it over with it, face up to the disappointment of not getting tickets instead of waiting in expectation.

Hyde Park festival holds thousands of visitors. Wheelchair platform holds 300. They won't make the platform bigger because they won't make so much money. Simple economics! But by providing the platform they are fulfilling their obligatory gesture towards the wheelchair. Hmmmm do they realise there is 11 million disabled people in the UK

Good job we are not all Celine Dion fans. Enough tickets for the "norms, not enough for the non norms" as my friend Kevin would say

I need a clever person work out percentages here. Tickets available v population v wheelchair users v platform spaces

Aside from my moaning here about the injustice of it all, my boys came good. Not happy about the situation at all we had a WhatsApp conversation and I realised how much this meant to them that I could be with them. And so Christopher contacts the ticket sellers AXS and explains our situation to them. They are really helpful and offer a complimentary ticket for a PA on the ground. We decide this is the best option even though it would mean I wouldn't be able to see and in my head I would be a small person surrounded by thousands of people standing around looking towards a stage. However, I then spoke to my Trelorian friends Kev and Janet who tell me it would be ok. This is a festival after all not just a two hour concert. There will be massive screens around the park and even though we couldn't see the stage we could find a position to park ourselves where we could watch one of the screens. We are still getting all the atmosphere of the event, just not view.

Ok so it's a compromise, but then we are used to that.

So for all of those people out there with your Celine Dion or whatever else tickets, next time you want to say "You're so lucky you get to park anywhere you want, (it isn't true, there are still regulations to be adhered to) or must be great to get paid just for being disabled" - spare a thought.... I'm not just one click away from getting to be equal.

A guide to flying and other holiday dilemmas

Flying when you can use crutches has its advantages and disadvantages. Walking down the aisle to your designated seat is awkward as they are generally narrow and designed for people with two feet side by side and not two feet side by side being flanked by a crutch either side. I had to do a kind of sideways manoeuvre. On the plus side I could get to the toilet. Annoyingly though cabin crew liked to take the crutches of me and put them overhead for safety reasons which meant pressing the buzzer and waiting for someone to give them back. On returning to my seat I would try to hide them under the seat in front and hope the crew forgot about them.

So this is how it happens in case anyone reading this is contemplating flying with a wheelchair user or indeed is the wheelchair user for the first time.

Most Airports and airlines follow a similar routine. Sometimes when you book the flight there will be a number to ring to discuss your requirements. They make ask you some questions about the size and weight of the chair. They may send you a form that needs to be filled in. Some airlines will give you at this point your seat number but if not it will be allocated at the check in desk.

Never turn up at an airport without having made it clear that one of you party is physically disabled. I have arrived at Stanstead Airport to board a Ryan Ait flight to Eindhoven and they claim they hadn't been pre-warned. I've being doing this a long time so I'm pretty confident I would have. This was back in the days when this airline would charge you £10 to use one of their wheelchairs. They said they couldn't help us as they hadn't been told and that if I still wanted to board the plane Graham would have to get me up the steps from the runway. They couldn't help due to health and safety. Their health and safety obviously, not ours! As he hauled me up those steps onto the plane, passengers were watching from the window. Most embarrassing, they were probably thinking we were going to delay their flight.

Once you get to the airport having pre warned them to expect you if you're lucky someone   spots you and you are taken from the queue to the front! Ignore the knives in your back from the passengers waiting. They will get their turn and the plane won't be taking off without them. Unless they are real knives of course!

Your wheelchair will be tagged. Don't let them put the tag on the hand rim of your wheel. Its really annoying. Let them put it on the footplate or main frame. You will be asked if you can walk up to the plane or up the steps if required or if, once on the plane you can leave your chair at the entrance and walk to your seat. Now don't ever be proud and say yes if this is going to cause you a problem. There is nothing worse than being stuck behind someone who says yes they can walk to their seat but forget to mention it may take some time. Remember there may be 200 people behind you. If you find it difficult say so now.

Once your tagged you may be asked to go to a designated spot to notify the assistance people that you are there. They will check on their list to make sure they have your name and the correct flight details. At this point you can choose to stay near to the assistance folk and wait or you can go for a wander and they will tell you what time to go through to departures. It doesn't always happen like this, sometimes you don't get to speak to the assistance people until you have passed through departures. Sometimes you may have to do it both times.

On passing through departures again you may be plucked from the queue and taken to the front. You will load any bags you're carrying into trays and because everyone has to pass through a security sensor you won't be able to do that as your chair will set of the alarms. Instead you have to be hand searched. A quick run up and down your back and legs and the chair gets checked with a special stick to ensure you're not carrying drugs in your wheels or something.

Ok so it's time to go back to the assistance team again if you have strayed from their sight. They will escort you down to the boarding gate where your chair is checked to make sure it's not lost its tag. So we are now ready to board. If the aircraft has a passenger boarding bridge then your assistance person or persons if required will push you down to the plane. You leave your chair at this point and if you have a wheelchair cushion I wouldn't recommend leaving it with the chair. It may get lost along the way. Carry it onto the plane with you. If you have opted to walk to your seat all well and good at this point but if you're not able to then they will be well prepared and have an aisle chair for you to transfer to. It's a bit like those ones you see sometimes in

189

ambulances. They strap you in and tip you back and reverse you along to your seat. If you're not able to transfer into your seat unaided then they will lift you.

If your plane is one where passengers embark from the tarmac up a flight of stairs then there will be an ambulift which is a bit like an ambulance but with a lift that takes you up to the opposite door to the one where the other passengers will be coming through. Beware these lifts can have slippy floors so I wouldn't advise you leaving your chair and walking until you are safely at the door of the plane. Once onboard it's time to get settled. Mostly the arm of the chair will lift up and its just a case of sliding across from the aisle chair but on some plains for whatever reason known best to them they don't. For me this makes it awkward and I have to be lifted over the arm into my seat.

There are certain seats they won't let you have. You will never be given a seat next to an emergency exit. To put it bluntly you will be in the way in the event of an evacuation as they assume, quite rightly I'm sure, that you can't just get up and run with the rest. They prefer you to have the aisle seat as it just makes it easier for them getting you in and out of it.

At this point your precious wheelchair is taken away and placed in the hold with the rest of the luggage. Generally speaking they aim to pre-board disabled passengers. This is ok as it means you're not jostling along with the other passengers trying to find their seats. It can be done calmly and at your own pace. They won't let the others on until you are settled.

People say "you're so lucky you get to board the plane first" What they never say is "you're so unlucky you have to wait until everyone is off the plane before you can get off" No one ever seems to notice that I am on the plane a good time longer than they are.

Of course it doesn't always work that way. Sometimes, if they have had a mad influx of us then the ambulift may not be available and you have to wait until it's free. It might be that several planes are departing or landing at roughly the same time. In this circumstance you can find that everyone else is already seated and waiting.

Disembarking? It really is just the same in reverse. You wait until everyone else is off the plane and then the assistance will come and get you. Now there are two advantages to this. Usually this means they have had time to find your own wheelchair and you can transfer straight away back into it. The other advantage is that by the time you get to baggage reclaim most of the other passengers will have collected their cases and it won't be as busy. Again if there are several planes with persons needing assistance taking of or landing at around the same time this can take a little longer but the good news is you won't be left alone. Someone from the cabin crew has to stay with you. If they haven't managed to get your own chair to you, then they will use an airport chair to get you back into the building while they go and look for yours.

No matter how hard I try to ensure that my trip is going to be snag free sometimes I hit a wall. The thing is we have to rely on the person who has deemed the accommodation to be suitable actually knows what they are talking about. Saying "yes it should be" isn't really good enough.

I searched on Trip Advisor for accessible apartments in Tenerife a couple of years ago. I found what appeared to be perfect. It had positive reviews and I was fairly confident. Right on the edge of the harbour in Los Cristianos and a reasonable price too. The apartment was on the top floor but had a lift. I emailed the owner and asked about the bathroom and the doorways. Yes he said the doorways were wide enough and he knew this for a fact because wheelchair users had stayed there before. Now wouldn't you think that by now I wouldn't be fooled by the claims of someone who clearly was just trying to sell me a two week booking?

Yes there was a lift. It had literally just enough space to fit my wheelchair in. Graham couldn't even get in and so every time we went out we had to meet in the foyer. Second issue was the bathroom. The doorway wasn't wide enough to get my chair in. Now had I still been a part time crutches user this wouldn't have been an issue but I'm not. So here is how we overcame the problem for the whole two weeks.

Take small chair from patio area and put just inside the bathroom door. Wheel up to bathroom door. Hitch across from wheelchair to chair. Ok so now I'm in the bathroom. To get to bath/shower transfer onto toilet. Lift chair and place next to bath. Transfer from toilet back onto chair again and then from there into bath. Simple but exhausting! I can only assume that when wheelchair users have stayed there before, they had been able to walk a little.

It's a common problem that some will make an assumption that all wheelchair users are the same which is I guess what happened in this case. I gave some feedback to him and he said he would take it on board and refurbish the bathroom. I don't know if he did. I don't really want to take the risk of booking again just in case.

If I'm booking a hotel in the UK, not for a holiday but for overnighters like when visiting London I will always go for Premier Inn or Travelodge because they are the two chains that I trust to get it right and the two that allow me to select an accessible room without the need to make any phone calls. No fuss, straight forward online booking.

Other hotel chains will show that they have accessible rooms but you still have to make that call to see if they have the availability.

Having sung the praises of the two mentioned above even they don't get it always right. A group of friends from my Treloar days met up in London to attend a memorial service. We selected a Premier Inn that had enough accessible rooms to accommodate all of us that were staying over the weekend. Graham wasn't coming with me so it was more important than ever that my room was adequate. My friend Beverley was also travelling alone. In both of our rooms whilst the bathroom lived up to all expectations the bedroom area had been poorly planned. If Graham had been with me, then not so much a problem but they had left very little room on one side of the bed. There was barely enough for a person to access the bed from, let alone a wheelchair. Most physically disabled people that I know, have a good and a bad side. Transferring for me, for example is always easier leading with my left side. If you can't get your chair round to the side of the bed you want then it can be difficult particularly if you are travelling alone. In addition to this, they had placed bedside lights on with side of the bed which were turned on and could only be turned off by the switch on the actual light. So picture this. Get into bed from the wrong side and then have to hotch across the bed to get to the lamp to switch it off. I can only surmise that the planners have made the assumption that the disabled person will always have a companion with them. I expect space is usually the reason for this kind of design.

Graham and I often stay at London City Airport Travelodge as it gives easy access into London to Jonathon's flat. Although I always request a double room, on the last two occasions we have been given the same room with twin beds. When Graham queried this with the evening receptionist her reply was "Well its twin beds because it's an accessible room" So there I am poised on the point of a complaint to Travelodge that they should not be making an assumption that disabled people require twin beds and don't sleep in double ones. But then, Graham queried it the following morning with the daytime receptionist who said he didn't know why accessible rooms have twin beds, when their website advertises all their rooms have king size double. Fortunately the Duty Manager was there and shecame to his rescue. She explained that although they were twin beds in that room, they could be hooked together to form a double, but the benefit of having twin beds was that they could be moved around to allow access from either side as is the preference of the disabled person! Gold star to Travelodge!

Both of these hotel chains do put a lot of thought into other nice touches. With low down dress rails, lower light switches and even "Crotch Height" spy holes in the doors. In the bathrooms most will have either sliding doors or extra wide bathroom doors. One gripe from a friend who is an amputee is that he finds showers hard to negotiate and would prefer a bath but the majority of

194

accessible bathrooms have wet rooms. This is more so in newer or refurbished bathrooms as some of the older ones do still have baths.

Of course, all hotels that offer disabled facilities will also have designated parking spaces as near to the door as possible as long as the "norms" have not parked in them.

Graham and I had a holiday to Malta. When we arrived quite late our hotel room wasn't ready and to be honest they gave that look that people give you when they realised they have messed up. We requested wheelchair friendly room and they had either forgotten or simply overlooked it. We were told that if we accepted a smaller room, they would move us the next day. After waiting for a while the following day the tour rep went to speak to reception for us and we were told we had been upgraded to a deluxe room. To be fair it was lovely and far superior to the pokey little room we had stayed in the night before.

The rep told us about the tours she had to sell us and we asked about the accessibility of each. She convinced us that getting on and off the coach would not be an issue so we booked a night tour of Malta, a trip to Gozo and a trip to the Craft shops.

With great difficulty I boarded the coach for the night trip much to the obvious impatience of the tour guide. A few days later we were ready for our trip to Gozo. Back onto a coach and then a ferry across from Malta. During the ferry journey the rep approached us and as tactfully as she was able to, she said that in Gozo there would be a lot of getting on and off the coach and she felt this would be too much for me. What she really meant was, she was on a tight schedule and I was too slow. She agreed to lay on a taxi at the company's expense so that we could follow the coach. When we returned to the hotel we asked for our money back for the third trip. Reluctantly she paid it and we used a private taxi to take us to the craft shops. The rep saw us there and she wasn't happy with the taxi driver for some reason and they ended up shouting stuff that we didn't understand. And the moral of the story? Beware Holiday Reps are there to sell you stuff and they really don't care if it's suitable of not.

The Toilet Connoisseur!

I have for a long time considered myself to be a connoisseur of *accessible* toilets. I don't like the phrase "Disabled Toilet" as I think this implies that the toilet is out of order. As in, it has been disabled. Accessible says to me that it is accessible to all. Over the last few years there have been massive improvements and availability to these facilities. A RADAR key is a skeleton key that can open any toilet that has the RADAR lock.

"The Royal Association for Disability and Rehabilitation, which is now Disability Rights UK, worked in partnership with Nicholls & Clarke, the inventors of the RADAR lock and together they created the National Key Scheme (NKS). The first RADAR locks were fitted in 1981 to help keep accessible toilets free and clean for disabled people.

Before RADAR locks were introduced, many establishments locked the accessible toilet themselves which meant that disabled people could only use the toilet on request. It also sometimes seemed to be the case that the key couldn't be located by the staff member, or the person who had it wasn't on duty that day. Fortunately, the introduction of the NKS meant disabled people could now use the toilet without having to ask someone if they could be let in"

Ok so the thing is this. Who do they consult when designing and installing one of these facilities? My biggest bug bear is the mirror. I think it's admirable that usually a mirror is provided but why is it that many of them you can't see from wheelchair height? A wide doorway is of course essential and handrails are most helpful but often the hand dryer will be a wheel away from the washbasin. This means that after washing my hands, I then have to wheel over to the dryer. I dry them and then put my hands back on my now wet wheels. Having said all of this I am most grateful that so many places now provide an accessible toilet so that I can go out with peace of mind that there will be one somewhere nearby. In a pub in London with Graham and the boys, I took my RADAR key and found the toilet. Unfortunately, I then had to move a table of young lads out of the way to get the door open! Fantastic that this lovely pub had one, but it was so small that the door had to be opened outwards. The space inside literally gave enough room for a toilet and my chair side by side. On the whole though, accessible toilets are adequate. That's if they aren't being used as storage space or changing rooms by the staff.

Recently we stayed at a Travelodge which had a lovely big spacious room with low mirror and handrails, shower seat, shower controls easily reachable. What I was puzzled about though was the positioning of the Emergency pull cord. It was just inside the door next to the light pull cord. So if I slipped in the shower, or fell off the toilet the cord was about eight feet away.

Occasionally we like to go camping. It takes the stress out of worrying about doorways! We always check that the camp site has accessible facilities and usually they will allow us to take the pitch as near to the facilities as possible. In 2018 we booked into a campsite for a week in Suffolk. Everything was checked out beforehand on their website and a quick phone call confirmed that we would be allocated one of their "Reserved for Disabled Pitches" On arrival we were shown to our pitch which literally was opposite the accessible shower and toilet. Experience has taught Graham and I to never take anyone's word for it until we have checked for ourselves. And so before the tent was set up, he went to check. Yes there was a ramp up to the door - tick. Yes there were handrails - tick. Yes even a low mirror - tick. However, the shower had a 12cms up and over step to be negotiated in order to get to the shower chair and shower - No tick. There was no way I was going a week without a shower so we spoke to the receptionist. She told us there was another shower block that we could use but it was at the opposite end of the campsite in a different field. We did stay the week but it was a mighty trek everyday!

Knowing your audience and other such matters

I don't know why some comments can be offensive and others funny. If a comment is upsetting is it the fault of the deliverer or the receiver?. Same goes if it's funny.

Here are some examples of things that have been said to me.

Health visitor when my firstborn was a baby. "I don't want you to worry but I think your baby will be slow to walk as he won't be able to copy you"
Ignorant and stupid.

Son Jonathon when about three years old - "Mum, I wish you weren't in a wheelchair," pause for heart wrenching moment. "You're always in the way of the Telly"
Funny and cute

Job interview "Oh, I'm sorry I didn't realise you were somewhat disabled"
Ignorant - so just makes me think it's obviously an issue or why is he apologising.

Hairdresser - "So why are you in a wheelchair? Oh Spina Bifida, you're so lucky to still be with us" followed by "My mum said my dad had that but I didn't believe her"
Just plain stupid.

Male Work colleague "So how do you get in and out the bath"
Odd? Why was he thinking about me in the bath!!!

Work colleague "If you come past me again I'll let your tyres down"
Not funny, boring. Heard it many times

Work colleague "Watch out, abnormal load coming through" or "Obstruction in carriageway"
Funny, because of the person who delivered it. He was making a mock attempt at being offensive - know your audience

Work colleague "If you need any help just stand up and shout"
Funniest part about this was the embarrassment he felt afterwards and his attempts to cover it up.

When starting work for the Police I had to go along with the other recruits to the stores to be measured for uniform. Stores lady looked at me and said "So how am I meant to measure you"
She was clearly thinking out loud

Friend "You're so lucky you can park anywhere"
Not true but wish it was

Man in pub "Brrrm Brrrm, watch me toes!"
Oh dear, so original

Man in pub "Watch out, it's Stirling Moss"
Never heard that before - Much

Another common question I'm asked is, "Is your husband in a wheelchair too!?
It wouldn't be an issue if he was, but would you approach a non-disabled person and ask "Is your partner a norm too?

Optician when discussing different finishes on my new glasses "Now I know you don't drive dear" and when I said "actually I do" her reply whilst patting my hand was "Oh well done you"

Ignorant and small minded

I telephoned a campsite earlier this year as I couldn't tell from their website whether their toilets would be able to accommodate a wheelchair. Yes the man said, but you would need to leave your chair outside to be able to shut the door.

Needless to say, I didn't stay there.

A singer in a bar in Tenerife - She came over to chat to us after her set. "So are you two a couple" "yes" we said. "So are you able to have sex and everything?"

No words are available from me for this

My Sister-In-Law   If you weren't disabled you could have a corner suite in this room.

This actually made sense but was still funny

There are some phrases and references that I'm not keen on.

Wheelchair Bound…..

"Bound" One definition in the dictionary is to walk or run with leaping strides???

Ok try again

"Something that is certain to happen" - well it certainly happened otherwise I wouldn't be writing this. Hmmm

"State of being constrained or tied" Yes that must be the one. That is where we get the phrase "Wheelchair Bound" from.

The thing is I'm neither constrained nor tied in the literal sense. I prefer to say I am a permanent wheelchair user. This is in the hope that whoever I'm speaking to understands that I am not able to walk at all.

Carer is another one.

A lot of places such as theatres and entertainment attractions will only charge the disabled person and not the "Carer" I went to Wimbledon this year with my Son and we only had to pay for 1 ticket as the "Carer" was free. He isn't my carer, he is my Son and my chosen companion for the event. So I would like to see companies changing their wording from "Carer" to "Companion" which would cover all bases in my opinion.

I attended an event called "HER DAY" which was all about empowering women in the workplace. Two Leicestershire Police Equality Officers, myself and Sarah who is the admin assistant in the Equality Office. Sarah is blind and had her assistance dog Rufus with her.. There were various stalls and exhibitions. We signed ourselves up for a session of mindfulness therapy. About a dozen or so people sitting around in a semi circle listening to a lady talk about well being, etc. Now she had rightly spotted that amongst our group I was in a wheelchair and Sarah was blind. All was going well until she said "Now those of you that can stand up, do so now" Ok; this would have been acceptable if she hadn't given me one of those "I'm sorry you're in a wheelchair" looks. Then she approached one of my colleagues and whispered to her, "Could you look after the blind lady please" Why whisper, and why mention "blind" lady. Sarah is not deaf. There were a few shocked faces, but mostly a lot of giggling going on instigated by Sarah herself.

It's not that anything malicious is meant, it's just that some people don't think before they speak. I call it their filter. What is worse than actually saying stuff is when they have the filter but it has a delay? The words start to come out and then they either stop…. And quickly try and change what they were going to say, or they say it anyway and then make things worse by apologising. "Do you want to come roller skating with us?"

Can become, "Do you want to come …..Wait for filter to kick in…..and watch us roller skating"

Or "OMG I'm so sorry, I didn't mean to upset you by asking you to come roller skating when you can't even skate" They then proceed to tell everyone else about the massive gaffe they have just made.

"Take a seat" is a phrase you will often hear in a waiting room. Love this one as it works one of two ways. Either the speaker will remain oblivious and carry on because at the end of the day it's just a phrase. It never means literally *take a seat* as this would mean they would forever have to replace the chairs. *Or* they panic as soon as they have said it and they never make eye contact with you for your remaining time in the room in case you are offended. Obviously the former is preferable. Of course the other option is "Just wheel yourself over there" and then they deserve to be a little smug at how well they handled the situation.

I don't think I am over sensitive about people. The thing that upsets me and I am maybe more sensitive about is situations. Such as the hassle with booking hotels, being turned away because of accessibility issues, wheelchair not fitting through doorways ETC So comments by individuals generally are ok and on the whole amusing. Let's face it, if they weren't I wouldn't be writing this book. If I'm talking about myself I will say "I walked to the shops" never "I wheeled to the shops" So if you asked me to go for a walk, without correcting, apologising or blushing with embarrassment then it's all good. It means you are looking at me as a person, not seeing the wheelchair as any kind of issue that needs to be highlighted. There is nothing worse, however, than someone being offended on my behalf.

Once at work a photographer came to take photos as the new department was being officially opened. The photographer saw me and asked if he could take a picture of me "at your desk *with your wheelchai*r" I did wonder if he meant as opposed to being seductively draped across the desk. A colleague overheard this and complained to management. I had to reassure them that I was not offended in any way. I could see what they were trying to achieve by showing what a diverse accommodating department it was. In fact another colleague also overheard and said "ask him if your duel heritage friend can be in the picture too" I get bored by strangers asking "Have you got a licence for that" "Hope you stick to the speed limit" "Look out, here come Stirling Moss" "Mind my toes with that thing" and similar. Not funny, not original. I smile politely as their efforts at wheelchair humour don't deserve any response from me and it only encourages them.

One colleague at work came over to me to ask a question, he put his hand on my shoulder and started to speak then said "Oh sorry, wrong person" I watched him cross the office and go to the only other physically disabled person in the room, Margaret…. Later he came back to me and apologised. I said "so all you were thinking was, you needed to speak to the disabled person, am I right?" And he admitted it and bought me some chocolate. Clearly a bigger deal for him than it was for me. Funnily enough the same guy did it again some months later, we met at a training event and he said "oh I heard you are changing jobs" "nope", I said "you've done it again, that's the other one" Now I could be offended but the humour of the situation far outweighed the annoyance.

The department I worked in, back in 2014 held some training days at a local David Lloyds Leisure Centre. It was compulsory for all staff to attend although on different dates due to the amount of people involved. We were given allocated seats on arrival. I found myself sharing a table with Margaret and my colleague and friend Sue who uses a walking frame. Was it a coincidence that the "disabled" were all placed on the same table? One of the organisers made a point of announcing to the room where the disabled toilet was whilst looking directly at us. Then during the course of the training the Sergeant in charge of the event pointed to our table and said "now everyone on that table stand up" I responded "Excuse me?" loved the look on his face when he glanced across and the penny dropped.

Is it wrong that I am amused at these faux pas? Graham says it's wrong because I'm encouraging them.

When Graham and I first officially became a couple he was living in a flat up one flight of stairs. I would go to his and climb the stairs. Enter and sit down breathlessly, where he would smile at me and say "Come on, we're going out now" You see the thing with Graham is that he just doesn't see the disability. He forgets that there are times when it's going to be difficult or just not going to work. He wanted to go on a sea fishing trip in Tenerife. I thought ok, this could be fun. He was positive there was no issue and showed me the boats.   Ok, so when he showed me the boats in the harbour the tide was in and the boats were raised to just below the pier. It's a challenge for anyone to walk across a gang plank to get on a small boat. It's almost impossible with crutches or a wheelchair. But we did it. When we got back however, the tide was out and the gang plank lay at 45 degrees to the pier. The boat owner gave me a most undignified fireman's lift. If he hadn't I would have had to wait for the tide to come back in. Couldn't rely on Graham doing it, he was too busy laughin

Another time, he suggested parascending. We bought the tickets and again, it was a case of waiting for the tide to be at its highest. We waited for a call and the following morning made our way back to the harbour. I have to say this was one of the most exhilarating experiences. Strapped into harnesses we went tandem and flew high above the sea. I was a bit concerned that the men on the boat that was pulling us had stopped looking up. I thought how will they know if we fall into the sea? We didn't of course. I loved it so much we did it again the next time we were there.

It's not the same !!

I have spent quite of bit of time in Central London. My sons, Jonathon and Christopher live and work there and husband Graham's hobby is Metal Detecting. He has a permit from the Port of London Authority to detect

206

on the Thames foreshore. Anyway, this entails a lot of DLR and Tube negotiating. Transport for London have helpfully included on their maps which stations have full step free access, although of course the DLR is proud to claim that all their trains and stations are wheelchair accessible.

I don't use the buses. I don't like the bit where all the passengers are held up while the ramp is engaged allowing me to board. Impatient passengers can give mean stares. They take umbrage if they have to move their Child's pushchair to allow a wheelchair into a designated space. It does mean quite a bit of planning to get from A to B. Jonathon is my main route planner. When we decide where we are going, he studies the map and gets me there. Sometimes it means going out of the way to walk back on yourself to get to where you want to be and I've never yet done it unaccompanied but if I lived in London permanently then I'm sure I would be able to manage it.

Travelling around London also involves a lot of Lift usage at stations etc. It puzzles me why some people prefer to stand and queue for a lift rather than walk up or down a flight of stairs. I'm not saying they don't have some hidden medical condition that makes stairs difficult but judging by how many times I've witnessed this I think it would be fair to say the majority are either plain lazy or don't understand that us wheelchair users just don't have a choice, whereas they do. I don't include people with suitcases, bicycles, pushchairs or other small children when I say this though. Some stations for example Green Park and Bank entail going up in one lift, changing lifts and going to another part of the station in another lift.

Anyway, so we find ourselves one day in St James Park having a picnic. A lady with small children started talking to me about the problems involved in negotiating London with a wheelchair. I said it's ok as long as you know which route to take. "Yes she said, I know exactly what you mean. It's the same with pushchairs" What? No it isn't. Wheelchairs are nothing like pushchairs. Yes admittedly they both have wheels and are used to transport a person but no, it's not the same. You can carry a child in a pushchair down a flight of stairs. Negotiating travel with a pushchair you have the option to take child out, carry them and fold up buggy or pushchair if needed. It's so not the same.

I challenge anyone to pick me up and carry me whilst at the same time transporting the wheelchair. Did I say all of this to this lady? No of course I didn't. She didn't mean offence, she wasn't rude, and she was merely being supportive in letting me know she understood. I could have corrected her but I smiled politely and agreed with her. I think perhaps she just wanted to make conversation and find a level of common interest. A means of communication about a topic we both understood.

We walked away. Christopher said "How is that ever the same?"

Cruising

When my parents used to take a cruise once a year they would come back with photos and tales of exotic lands and amazing experiences they had had. I always thought cruising wouldn't be practical for me though.

My only real experience of boats was a ferry from England to Spain as a child and once a school trip to Holland. I remembered them to have really high lips on the doorways that you had to step over. I couldn't envisage a cruise ship. I also thought that when the ship docked at each port everyone had to leave the boat and get on one of those tenders to get to the port.

I nearly got to find out in 2004 when mum and dad had booked to go on one but she had to cancel as she was in hospital having been diagnosed with breast cancer again. When visiting one afternoon she asked if Graham and I would be interested in going if they could change the booking. We were meant to be going to Malta later that year but I would cancel that if there was a cruise on offer. She convinced me it would all be perfectly wheelchair accessible. I went home and spoke to Graham. We agreed that providing we could both get the time of work then yes, we would love to. The next day I went to visit again and she told me that she had also mentioned it to my brother Chris and his partner Sue. Almost immediately Sue had contacted the cruise company and had the tickets transferred into their names. So that was that. A done deal and I didn't get to find out if I liked cruising.

After dad died and we had paid back Graham's sister Doreen, the extortionate Spanish Inheritance Tax plus other debts that we had from Tenerife we had a little money left over. During the London Olympics of 2012, two months after arriving back in the UK and me returning to work, I noticed my right leg, the one that had been the problem in Tenerife, was red and swollen. Graham took me to A & E at Leicester Royal Infirmary where it was suggested I had a DVT. Whilst we waited to be seen they took blood from me. An Orthopaedic doctor walked into the cubicle took one look at me and said "This lady has a broken tibia" – oh god, here we go again. I was sent for an X-ray and when I returned to the cubicle another dr came to see me. He said judging by the results of my blood test I should be dead! He asked another dr for a second opinion and they went away for a discussion. Re-appearing a short time later the dr then said I could go home with a splint on my leg and he gave me an appointment to go to the fracture clinic the following week. "But what about my blood?" I asked. Red faced the dr said "Oh that, sorry we got the results round the wrong way, you're not dead"!!!

I attended the fracture clinic the following week and saw an orthopaedic consultant called Mr Godsiff. He said the broken tibia would heal but he was more concerned about my knee. That was the bone that I had broken in Tenerife. It was my femur, just as above the knee joint. I was so fed up by this point I begged him to amputate the bloody thing. This leg was causing my so much trouble that I really thought I would be better off without it. He wouldn't agree to it. He said it would cause me more problems with balance etc. And so he suggested a total knee replacement which he believed would fix the problem. He would cut away the damaged part of the femur then insert a false knee joint that would have to be specially made as my bones aren't exactly standard design.

In February 2013 at Glenfield General Hospital I was admitted for the operation. It was a long, long operation lasting about six hours where they recycled my own blood back into my body rather than a standard blood transfusion. After the operation I had a couple more blood transfusions. The other patients on the ward having knee or hip replacements were allowed home once the physio was happy they could weight bare. This proved to be a tad tricky in my case. And so I stayed an extra few days just to be sure everything was ok. I was told not to attempt to weight bare for about six weeks but after that it should be safe. So we decided we could take a little holiday whilst I was covered by a sick note. Essential recuperation was my excuse.

We went to our nearest travel agent which was Co-Op travel and asked about holidays to America. I wanted to go to Las Vegas and we thought we would split up the long flying by visiting other places. The agent gave us some ideas and talked about suitable hotels. After about an hour we got a quote. Then Graham said, "Just to throw a spanner in the works, what about cruises" Another hour later we had details of a last minute Caribbean Cruise and Stay with Thomsons. Fly to Barbados then board the ship for a week. The second week would be spent at a resort in Barbados before flying back home. Perfect. We asked about accessible cabins obviously and the lady said she needed to make a phone call. It was a Saturday so the office she needed to speak to was closed. She said she wouldn't be able to confirm a suitable cabin until Monday. Monday morning she rang us. She still wasn't able to confirm an accessible cabin as it was now less than 14 days until departure. Apparently it's down to the Captain and crew to allocate cabins within the last 14 days and not the travel agent so it was out of their hands. She suggested we go ahead and book and then hope to get an accessible cabin once on board.

No, I don't think so.

What would happen if there wasn't one? Do we sleep on the floor in the Atrium (See I had been looking it up and I knew proper cruise ship words) There was no way we could take that chance. I got upset. I do every now and again when I think life is unfair or that I am being discriminated against. The point was that on the Saturday if that office had been open we would have been within the time constraint to book a cabin with Co-Op Travel.

Graham spent the next few hours on the phone ringing different companies, determined I would get my cruise. Eventually he spoke to a lady at P & O who said she had an accessible cabin on a shi p that was sailing from Barbados around the Caribbean for 14 nights leaving in 2 weeks time. Sold!

The lady from Co-Op travel did call back the next day to offer an alternative. I said, politely, "No thank you, we are sorted" She asked "May I ask how you have sorted it?" My reply was "Yes we booked with another company who don't discriminate.

Then there was a mad rush to buy suitable attire. Long frocks, cufflinks, dicky bows etc we were off flying to Barbados. It was a 10 hour flight and I didn't know then that long haul flights always have an aisle chair and a sort of disabled toilet. So I drank a minimal amount of liquid and packed a she-wee just in case.

The cruise on the Azura was just amazing. I loved every minute of it. We didn't understand about the protocols of the dining experience so we had opted for set dining which meant we always ate at the same table for two. The alternative was freedom dining where you could choose from the different restaurants on board or just opt for the 24 buffet.

The cabin we had was big and had a balcony and the bathroom was a wet room where the shower chair I had requested was already in situ. At each port it was a simple act of leaving the ship by ramp where the stewards insisted on taking charge and have a walk into whichever town it we were docked at. All P & O had asked of me was the dimensions of my wheelchair and if I had any dietary requirements. We were sent by their special services department detailed information about ports we would be visiting and excursions and which were wheelchair friendly should we wish to book. It was all fabulous and far exceeded my expectations. Not since Florida and Disneyworld had I ever experienced a more inclusive, disability friendly holiday.

Shortly after returning from that cruise, I was in the bathroom at home (As I've said, it's always in a toilet) when I transferred onto the toilet and heard a familiar crack. As it was bedtime I decided not to say anything to Graham and I went to bed carefully!

Next morning I knew something wasn't quite right and I told Graham that I thought something was wrong with my leg. I could feel my femur sort of moving around so we went back to A & E. Another x-ray confirmed my femur had snapped just above the new knee joint. Right so, here's what had happened – concentrate, its technical! The bones in my legs are not straight. If I stood up my legs would be oval shaped like an egg, not straight up and down, so when they fitted the metal work for the knee replacement it wasn't a good enough fit for the cement to set. The metal frame for the knee had come away taking the femur with it, causing it to snap. I was admitted to Leicester Royal Infirmary and waited for someone to make a decision about what to do. After visits from several different specialists finally one came to see me who said he thought he could mend me. Mr Bogahdia was a specialist in treating bone cancer patients and he said that he could insert some sort of metal construction to save my leg. It was like the meccano that my brother used to play with. A metal bracket with holes in that was fixed to my femur by wrapping wire around and around it. He said that if it failed then the only other option was amputation. That was in 2013 and so far it seems to have worked, but they do keep checking once a year for metal fatigue which is comforting.

Yes I still have daily pain, and I am less agile that I was before the whole broken leg in Tenerife incident but it's ok. Part of the experience of being me!

Anyway, having loved the first cruise so much we did another one in August 2013 around the Mediterranean. My posh frocks deserved another outing, as did Graham's tuxedo. Again with P & O and again I absolutely loved the confidence of knowing it was all going to be accessible and completely ok. One day when we had docked in Sardinia I wasn't able to leave the ship because they were using a tender to get passengers to the island and it wasn't safe for wheelchairs. I and all the other wheelchair users congregated around a table in the bar and discussed disabilities! It turned out that they all had categories of disability according to the level of paraplegia! I felt a bit left out, I was the only one who had been born this way and so I didn't have a category that I knew of!

After that we took a three night mini cruises with P & O to Bruge, Belgium and decided that for a Christmas present that year we would take whichever of our children wanted to go. In April 2014 we took my Chris and Graham's daughter Kerry and sons Neil, Ross and

Wayne. We needed two cars to get to Southampton and on the way I got a puncture in my Motability Ford Fiesta. We had stopped at Sutton Scotney Services and I drove over a pothole. The RAC couldn't guarantee getting to me in time to get to the ship for boarding. I panicked. But Graham reckoned we would all fit in his car which was a Vauxhall Zafira Estate. And so we continued our journey with seven people, plus luggage, plus wheelchair for the last 20 miles of the journey, squashed but relieved. To keep the cost down we opted for an inside cabin rather than a balcony. It was smaller than we had had before but still good enough for our needs. We just had no idea about whether it was night or day!! Or maybe that was down to the alcohol.

Fast forward to 2016 and we were ready to cruise again. We tried Thomsons again as they offered an unlimited drinks package which appealed to us. I set about trying to book a 10 day cruise around the Canaries. Yes we could have flights to Tenerife and board the ship from there. No problem. Let's face it I knew my way round Tenerife Sur Airport. So far so good! Then the agent on the phone said she couldn't book me an accessible cabin because the spreadsheet was locked. She suggested I call back later. I did. And again and again over the course of several days and each time I was told the spreadsheet was either locked or inaccessible or being updated. One day they told me that the staff from the night before hadn't released it to the day staff.

In frustration we gave up. Sorry Thomsons you are not getting my money.

After a bit more Googling we found an American Company where we could fly to New York and cruise to the East Caribbean. It was a reasonable price and included an unlimited drinks package. We booked a cruise only deal and I sorted out flights with Virgin and a Days Inn not far from JFK airport to stay the night before. The price of the hotel included a free transfer to our hotel. Unfortunately after negotiating our way around the huge JFK airport we discovered that none of the transfer buses were accessible. We rang the hotel to explain this and they advised us to get a cab. Retracing our steps back again on the opposite side of the airport we found a yellow cab taxi rank and we managed to get a "Handicap Transfer" cab. On arriving finally at the Days Inn the receptionist was most apologetic and reimbursed us the cab fare. A porter was called who showed us to our room. Our non-wheelchair accessible room! Back down to reception were we showed the receptionist our booking confirmation from booking.com clearly stating what was required, an Accessible room. By this time it was about 2.30am to our body clocks and bitterly cold with snow on the ground. The porter tried again and this time we were shown to an adequately accessible one. The following morning, the hotel receptionist sorted us with a taxi to the airport. We explained we needed a fairly big one for the wheelchair and expected another yellow cab. Imagine our surprise when a beautiful black limousine complete with suit wearing chauffeur turned up.

As for the actual cruise itself, cruising with NCL was an entirely different experience to P & O. To begin with, they have a casual dress code. No formal black and white dressing up events and so no posh frocks needed. The majority of the passengers were Americans.

We met some lovely people who were fascinated to learn all about England and our heritage as one person pointed out, we have centuries of history and they don't

In the casino you could smoke! We were shocked and surprised but at least I had one very happy hubby. We made friends with a guy from California who introduced himself as "Fat Bastard" He handed us his business card "Fat Bastard, It's a way of life" I had to look twice, yes is really did say "Fat Bastard". We couldn't argue with him about the fat bit. He, Richard, was a big, big, man who could be found every day holding court at the pool bar. Big, but a very happy and fun guy. Our stateroom was good with a window but no balcony. There were no issues with the toilet and wet room. The food wasn't bad but not quite up to P & O standards.

As we were sailing from New York in January, and it would take several days to get to the Caribbean, the first couple of days it was cold and a bit choppy but every day after that it became warmer and calmer until at last we had five days of beautiful Caribbean sunshine.

On the way back to New York however we got caught up in the aftermath of a storm in Nova Scotia. It was rough and they stopped everyone from going on deck. Any excuse to spend a couple of days in the Casino. Richard didn't gamble but he did smoke. As he couldn't get up to the pool bar where it was permitted, he sat in the casino until the manager told him he couldn't stay as he wasn't gambling and was asked to leave. It put a bit of a sour note on our last day to be honest. When we booked the cruise several months before it sounded ideal and then Graham said well if we are going all that way why not have a few extra days and go to Vegas.

It sounded simple and it would have been for a "normal couple" but by now I'm an expert in travel arrangements so I set about sorting out the flights with Virgin extended them for another five days to incorporate this extra little bit of holiday. Finding a flight to Las Vegas from JFK on the day the ship docked back into Manhattan was easy enough. It was a five hour flight so

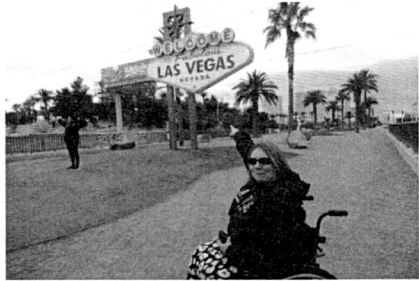
Fabulous Las Vegas

not too bad. It was a bit rocky as we were flying east to west inland. The more difficult task was sorting out flights that would get us back into JFK in time for our return flight to Gatwick with Virgin. It was a little more challenging even without booking all that wheelchair assistance. Hotels and McCarren International Airport in Vegas were really accessible as were the taxis. We really did have a *fabulous* time. Even when I made Graham walk about four miles from our hotel to see the famous "Welcome to the Fabulous Las Vegas" sign. Fremont Street in downtown Las Vegas had a restaurant called "The Heart Attack Grill Bar" and it had a set of scales outside. If you weighed more than 350lbs you ate for free!! We had to pay for storage at JFK so we didn't take all our cruise gear to Vegas and incur extra baggage charges. So from a disability point of view it all went to plan. The real challenge was getting over the jet lag on the return. Las Vegas is three hours behind New York and New York is five hours behind London. So in effect

218

we had an eight hour time difference to contend with. We left Vegas at 5.30am and flew to JFK where it was 1.30pm when we arrived. We flew from JFK at 6.30pm and arrived in London at 6.30am

It took about a week to get over it, it's not just the tiredness it's the disorientation. I could barely say my own name when I returned back to work a couple of days later.

By early 2017 we started talking about another cruise for January 2018. It would be a two year break. Again we booked with NCL for the same cruise. The difference was that this time we would let NCL do it all. Price wise it did actually work out cheaper. They booked us on Norwegian Air from Gatwick to fly the day before the cruise departure and into The Marriott Hotel Times Square with a Wheelchair accessible transfer bus. The following morning there would be a wheelchair accessible bus to transfer us to the Cruise Ship.

We nearly didn't go. Hurricanes Irma and Maria caused devastation across many Caribbean Islands including ones that we were due to visit. We waited to see if the trip would be cancelled by NCL before paying the balance in late November. They didn't cancel but the itinerary was changed. Then a week before both of us came down with the flu. A couple of days before the washing machine broke. Was someone trying to warn us not to go?

The assistance at Gatwick and the flight were fine. When we got to JFK there was an NCL rep waiting to greet us. He showed us the vehicle that had come to pick us up and apologised. He said "Don't worry, this won't be the one that collects you in the morning"

Well it was a wheelchair accessible vehicle in that it had a lift and clamps to keep the chair in place, just a bit old and tatty as was the driver. The taxi itself was adequate. The driver wasn't. It was a petrifying drive through the street to get into Manhattan. He drove fast and seemed to have no awareness of other vehicles sharing the road. We arrived at the hotel miraculously in one piece. The hotel looked impressive and we took the elevator to reception where we checked in and were shown to our room by a porter.

Yes I bet you guessed. It wasn't wheelchair accessible. No way would my chair fit through the bathroom door. And back to reception where we were moved to another room. Why does this keep happening we wonder? Is it the fault of NCL or The Marriot? We asked the receptionist why, when she saw me sitting there at "Crotch Height" did she not make the connection that we would need a Handicap room. The receptionist's response was "Well we didn't want to make an assumption"

After a good night's rest we waited for our new transport to take us to the ship along with two more British couples who were also being picked up by NCL. It was about an hour late and the NCL rep was most apologetic as we waited outside the hotel. My heart sank when the same guy with the same old tatty vehicle turned up. We all squashed in with our luggage. I had to hold onto one of the cases to stop it from rolling every time the driver braked. As we approached the port the driver slammed the brakes on so hard that I was nearly thrown from my chair. It was only the fact I was hanging onto a case that saved me.

The Stateroom was ok. No balcony or window but we got what we paid for. Our choice so can't really blame anyone for that mistake. The real problem was the passengers who had mobility scooters and parked them outside their cabins. Some were their own and others were ones they had hired from NCL. Now the rules clearly state that only mobility aids that can be stored in your stateroom can be taken on board. Anything bigger must be stored in designated spots. It's an obvious health and safety risk to block walkways. We complained that I couldn't get down the walkway to get to my cabin and were told it would be sorted. They were moved. The following day I couldn't leave the cabin for the same reason. The scooters were back. We complained over and over again and even took photos. Now I'm very happy for people who are able to leave their scooter at the door and walk inside but rules are rules.

This cruise was not a patch on the last time. Same ship, Norwegian Gem and same cruise company but the food was very bland and barely hot enough. In the buffet restaurant they had designated tables as priority for disabled passengers but this wasn't monitored and barely adhered to by other able bodied passengers. The ongoing problem with the scooter obstructions all led to it being a less that enjoyable experience.

The Islands we visited were lovely but whereas P & O always ensured accessible transfers if required, with NCL it was sort yourself out.

Towards the end I became unwell. I remained in the cabin for most of the last two days barely eating. Just sleeping and drinking water. On the last night I tried to take some paracetamol and was sick. Graham went to find our steward to ask for clean bedding and was told "Sorry we don't have any spare double duvets, we only have single ones" No spare bedding? Really? Well I suppose it was so near to the steward's end of shift and obviously a bit of an inconvenience.

We were quite relieved to get off that ship in the end. We had delayed the return flight by two nights to spend them in New York. My sons Jonathon and Christopher had flown out a couple of days before and were staying in the same hotel. Hotel Pennsylvania. I had booked us all tickets to see Chicago on Broadway and knew I had to kick this bug whatever it was.

Time for a little trivia I think - The Hotel Pennsylvania that I had opted for in Manhattan, the cheapest deal I could find, has the longest continuous use of a telephone number in New York. Can you guess? Of course it is "Pennsylvania 6-5000" the inspiration for a song recorded by Glenn Millar and then The Andrews Sisters.

We came out of the Port and looked for a taxi. We saw a Handicap bus and the driver waved to us. We got on board and he set off. We said where we wanted to go but the driver said somewhere else. "No" Graham said. "We need to get to Hotel Pennsylvania" The driver turned and looked at us. He asked if I was someone called Pauline. I said no. Then his phone rang and it was Pauline wanting to know where her taxi was. We had jumped into a taxi that someone else had pre booked. He turned around and took us straight back to the Port where we received a barrage of abuse from a very cross Pauline. The two days in New York were good with the boys, despite feeling so ill. On Sunday afternoon they contemplated leaving me in bed and pinching my wheelchair to go to the Theatre. I got a concession on the price as in the UK and could have 3 companions. So someone had to be in the chair!! But dosed up nevertheless I made it and as we approached the Theatre a lady came along and pushed people out of the way saying "Move please, Handicap person coming through" We should have checked out of the hotel Monday lunchtime but our flight wasn't until 10.30pm so Christopher rang reception and said we needed to pay extra to keep the room longer as I wasn't well.

By the time we got to JFK none of us were sure they would let me on the plane. I had a woolly hat pulled down and a scarf pulled up to cover me as much as possible so no one would notice. As soon as we got home Graham rang for a doctor who came and checked me over. As soon as she heard we has come from the Caribbean and been on a cruise ship she declared that I may have Legionnaires Disease or possibly Pneumonia. "She needs to get to hospital "Am I calling an ambulance or are you taking her"

At A& E I was given intravenous antibiotics. The Doctor said he could admit me so that they could keep topping me up or I could go home with a prescription for some industrial strength antibiotic tablets. It wasn't Legionnaires, it was a really bad chest infection that had the potential to turn to Pneumonia had it been left any longer untreated.

I wrote to NCL and gave them a list of my complaints. They addressed each one of my issues and said I could have a voucher for money of my next cruise. I refused and said I wouldn't be travelling with NCL again so they reimbursed me £400 which included a refund of the compulsory gratuities that we had to pay up front.

And that is cruising experiences so far. I want to do it all again but I think I will stick to P & O to be safe. I know there are equally good companies out there but I know where I am with them. My advice is do your homework and don't necessarily go for the cheapest option.

Treloarians on Tour

For a few years after leaving Treloars I stayed in touch with a couple of friends. Sally lived in London and we visited each other from time to time. In fact Sally borrowed my wedding dress from when I had married Eamon and wore it at her first wedding. That marriage lasted about as long as mine and so she burnt it! Can't say I blame her. Elizabeth who lived in Southampton came to Leicester and we went back to Treloars to visit together once. But eventually as we all moved on with our lives we drifted apart. To communicate with school friends who lived 100 plus miles away it meant writing, telephoning or just turning up at their door. Although that was just how it was before the internet and social media, the introduction of Facebook was the platform that reconnected so many of us.

I joined Facebook in 2009 and quickly old names and faces started to emerge. I learnt that two ex Trelorian friends, Kevin and Janet had married. Two other friends Roz and Ian who I knew had married now had a family. I made contact with Sally, Beverley and Marie but couldn't find Elizabeth. Other names and faces popped up and we began reconnecting. Eventually Elizabeth found me! Quite a challenge as my name had changed again since she has last seen me, she did well! Marie had married a guy called Roland and was living in London and it was so good catching up.

Someone then created a Facebook page, Trelorians - Where are they now? And gradually all the years faded away as more and more former Treloarians emerged. We swapped memories and anecdotes. Everyone had such tales of our time away from home.

Sadly there were far too many that didn't make it. Physical disability can take its toll and sometimes the body just says "That's enough"

Treloars, which since 1978 the year I left, had amalgamated the boys and girls schools into one, hosts a reunion at what was previously my Florence Treloar School. This site was now the location of Treloars School and Treloars College and what was previously the site of the Lord Mayor Treloar College in Froyle has been sold off as a development. The range of ages currently is from 2yrs right through to 25.

In 2015 I made the effort to attend one of these reunions and met with old friends that I hadn't seen in 37 years. There was just so much to catch up on and we simply didn't have enough time in those two days. It was also quite a shock to see how much the school had physically changed to accommodate the levels of disability being accommodated today, with much more need for hoists and staff far outnumbering students. After being told off at the reunion for being too noisy! we decided we would start our own spin off group. I began planning a meet up. Graham and I had a motor home so what I was looking for was a camp site that also had a B & B. Obviously the B & B needed to be wheelchair friendly. I telephoned a place I found on the internet called Honeysuckle Homestead in Dinton, Wiltshire. Elsie, Robin and their daughter Corina and husband Andy owned a small campsite and the B & B had been converted from a nursing home. I gave them a date we had in mind and reserved rooms for Sally, Beverly, Marie and Roland. Kevin and Janet would join us in the day time but not stay over as they lived in Amesbury, not too far away. Graham and I stayed in our motor home. We BBQ'd around the motor home. We had six wheelchairs amongst us and two walkers. Graham and Roland were run of their feet. It was a success so we decided to do it again towards the end of the summer as a couple had not been able to make it.

In September we all met up again at Honeysuckle. This time we were joined by Roz. Seven wheelchairs! We were growing. On our first visit in May Elsie and Corina had asked for input as to how they could make improvements to accommodate disabled guests. We gave them ideas and suggestions about grab rails, light switch height, positioning of toilet roll holders, making the bedroom door closures easier and of course ramps, based on our combined vast experience. Honeysuckle Homestead had one room that had a sliding door on the

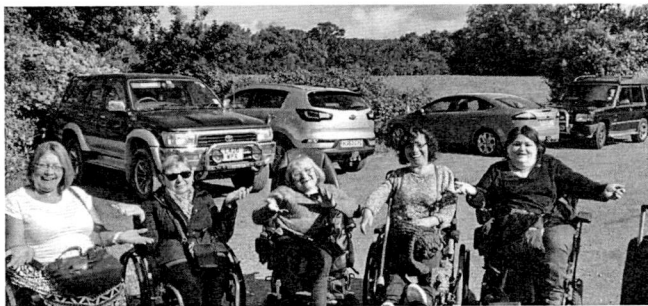

Honeysuckle Homestead Treloarians On Tour, Dinton, Wiltshire 2015

bathroom, a seat in the shower and a raised toilet seat but the rest of the rooms were standard en-suite bedrooms. They kindly let us make use of the B & B breakfast room in the evenings to gather around and chat when it got too cold to sit by the motor home.

We decided on a change of location and although it's really not easy finding suitable accommodation for one wheelchair, the real challenge is to accommodate a group such as ours. Nevertheless in 2016 Beverley found us a purpose built venue. "The Beamsley Project" in Skipton, Yorkshire. Not so many of us this time but still a good time was had by all. Roz, Ian, Dean (Ian's brother also ex Trelorian), Chris (Ian and Dean's cousin – Yes another ex Trelorian), Beverley, myself and Graham. The facilities were purpose built as a holiday retreat for disabled people and had hoists and other specialist equipment. We didn't need any of that of course. We were Trelorians we could cope with anything as long as the doorways were wide enough and there was a lift if it wasn't all ground floor. The kitchen was amazing. With adjustable height worktops and appliances, including a cooker and hob that had winder handles so that you could raise or lower them. This allowed preparing and cooking at a safe and comfortable height. Roz took charge of breakfast with the appliances lowered to wheelchair user height. She was in her element. Then Graham would wind them back up again to cook the evening meal at standing height.

We each had an allotted task and Chris took charge of dishwasher loading duties. For fun on the last day we asked him what the dishwasher was called as he was clearly quite fond of it. He replied without hesitation "Stephanie" I have no idea why I should remind him of a dishwasher but it amused everyone else! Three wheelchairs and four walkers!

The following year we had a different kind of break. We all met up in London in October 2017 for a memorial service to remember the haemophiliacs that had passed away due to the scandal of the contaminated blood in the 1980's.

I won't go into too much of the details of this scandal as I don't think I have enough knowledge to give it the justice it deserves. But I will explain as best I can. Haemophilia is a blood disorder that prevents the blood from clotting. It is caused by an Inherited Genetic Mutation which mainly affects males. This inherited alteration to the DNA sequence explains why several males from one family can be affected, i.e. brothers and cousins. The Haemophiliac boys could be given an injection of a product known as factor VIII which replaced the need for hours of blood transfusion. But the stock in Britain of this product couldn't keep up with the demand and blood started to be imported from America where donors would be paid for their blood. This attracted donations from drug users, prisoners and prostitutes amongst others. All 89 boys were found to have been infected with Hep B and Hep C. 64 of them contracted HIV from imported contaminated blood. The way the news was broken to them was that they were called to the medical centre in groups of five. They were told that there had been a problem with the blood they had been given and one by one given the news was delivered as to whether they had HIV or not. They were told they may only have two to three years to live. Of the 2,500 infected patients in the UK that have passed away, 73 of them were Students from Treloars. In a nutshell it was a tragedy that should never have occurred and those boys still with us along with the families that were left behind are still fighting for justice. A public enquiry began in May 2019 that aimed to uncover how and why this scandalous catastrophe was ever allowed to happen.

And so it was that in London on a Saturday in October 2017 we were a party of seven wheelchairs and seven walkers who made our way to the Church to meet with others attending the memorial service. We must have posed an intimidating site as we made our way from the Premier Inn, Aldgate to the church on that Saturday morning. Normally I get walked into or tripped over but this time we couldn't be missed. People crossed the road rather than try and pass us. Of course we didn't go single file that would have just looked ridiculous. No, we were a mob on a mission. Jon, my son, was with me as Graham was off metal detecting that weekend. Amongst the throng were Richard (ex Trelorian) and his wife Vanessa. The service was very moving. The names of all those that had passed away was read out and families lit candles in remembrance

After the service we walked back towards the hotel to find somewhere to eat. We spotted a Greek restaurant and Richard went to ask if they could accommodate us all. They moved a few tables around and in we went. Part way through the meal, much to our surprise a woman came in carrying a portable cd player which she placed on a table. She switched some Arabic style music on and began belly dancing. I guess part of her act seemed to be to select one or two male diners and persuade them to dance with her. As we were the only table in there at that time her choice was a bit limited. Scanning our table with all its wheelchairs she needed to make a quick decision. She chose Richard as a safe option as he was sitting on a dining chair. Up he went to dance with her. She then did a quick check again amongst the mass of wheelchairs until she spotted and selected Jon. He was brave and stuck it out until she let him return to his seat.

It was a funny night watching them both attempting belly dancing. We were all in fits of laughter. Not so much at the dancing but more about the quandary that must have faced that belly dancer about who to choose without revealing the panic she must have been feeling

Kevin and Janet are music enthusiasts and attend as many concerts and festivals in a year as they can possibly fit in. Graham is a fan of SKA music so it made sense when Kevin suggested we get tickets for a SKA gig at the NIA Birmingham in May 2018. This was new to me. An outdoor concert! Roz and Ian came along and even though Roz and I only knew 2 of the songs from a whole 4 bands event, a fabulous

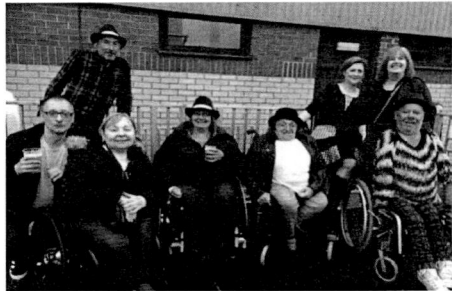
Ska - Birmingham May 2018

time was had as we viewed the acts from our special Wheelchair Viewing Platform. Sadly Pete Shelly, lead singer of Buzzcocks, died in December 2018 just months after appearing at this event.

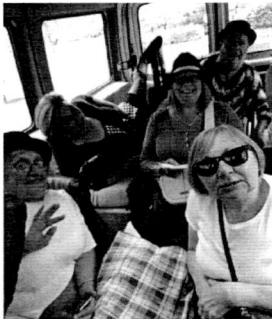
Treloarians Tour Bus!

Having had a break of two years from our reunion breaks in 2018 I thought I would have another go and faced a further challenge to find us all accommodation. We were growing in numbers every time. Graham and I had to travel to Somerset to get a car seat fitted

230

to the Renault Master adapted Vehicle we had bought to replace my Motability car. On the way back we stayed at a B & B called The Dark Barn Lodge. It was all ground floor and even though they only had 1 specifically designed room with wet room, the owner assured us that all the rooms and bathrooms could accommodate wheelchairs.

We returned home and put the suggestion to our Trelorian gang. Yes, good idea count me in was the response. I reserved all their available rooms for Marie and Roland, Kevin and Janet, Beverley, Roz and Ian, Dean and Linda, Richard and Vanessa and Elizabeth who had now also joined in. It was almost a complete take over. On the Saturday we were also joined by yet another ex Trelorian, Andy. We were now officially Trelorians on Tour. The group had grown again. However, the accommodation let me down on this return visit. I had spoken to the owners many times over the weeks before confirming the booking and they couldn't be more helpful. But when we all arrived I could sense there was something not quite right. Gone was the customer service that we had experienced on our first visit and I can only describe the owners as being people that really didn't want to be there or be inconvenienced with us being there.

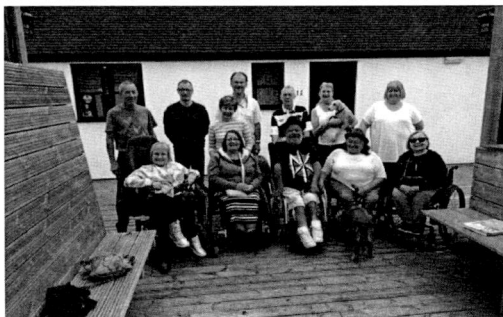

Dark Barn Lodge - Gloucestershire August 2018

231

Something just wasn't quite right.

Sometimes you just get that feeling. The car park was covered in gravel that had been there on our first visit but had looked as if it was only temporary and part of a refurbishment plan. Not small pieces but large stones. Wheelchairs and gravel don't go well together. It's virtually impossible to wheel across them without help in a manual or an electric chair. The owner said that he wasn't allowed to tarmac by the local council as it wouldn't be environmentally friendly. They had told me that before our stay they would be installing a type of roof in the courtyard which would be useful incase of inclement weather. On arrival there was no roof and all the plants in the planters in that courtyard, that had looked so pretty before, were dead.

Then we found out from the local pub that they were selling up which explained everything. We BBQ'd the first night and the second night we went to a pub for dinner. Graham had phoned the pub a couple of weeks before to check it was all "wheelchair friendly" and to reserve a table for 15 of us. You see, as I keep emphasising, it's all about the planning. Experience has taught us over the years that spontaneity rarely works. When we got there Graham, our designated scout, went in to check before we all piled in. Too many times we

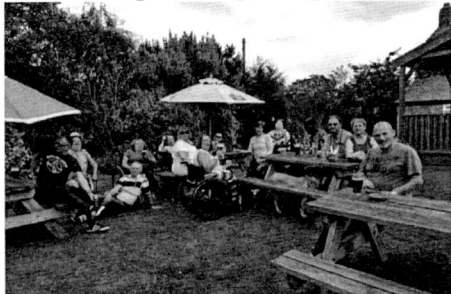

Treloarians in a pub!! 2018

232

have been promised things by people that just don't understand the difficulties that we can face. Our reserved table was perfectly set up for us all. They had allocated us a lovely private room where they had thoughtfully positioned all the tables into a rectangle which meant that we could all sit together.

Unfortunately there was a large step into this room!

Now whilst those of us with manual chairs could be helped up, there is no way an electric chair can be assisted in the same way as they are so heavy. Once the staff understood the problem the excuse was, that the person that Graham had spoken to when he made the booking on the phone, was on a day off and failed to pass on the message. After a lot of running round and head scratching by the staff with the other customers joining with suggestions and offers to help, a ramp was constructed from a couple of planks of wood! All sorted.

As I have mentioned previously Graham and I are Rocky Horror Show fans and we thought it would be fun to make a "Trelorians on Tour" mini break. Not everyone could make it, although Elizabeth's husband Liam had bravely joined the gang, so there were eight of us booked into the Premier Inn, Birmingham City Centre, Bridge Street which was about a ten minute walk (wheel, hop, skip or jump – take your pick) to the Alexandra Theatre where the show was performing. Big shout out to the Premier Inn staff that really went beyond expectations to provide us with amazing service and hospitality. Nothing was too much trouble for them. The accessible rooms with en-suite bathrooms were huge and there was adequate disabled parking. As it so happened, this also coincided with Birmingham Pride weekend and the whole of Birmingham seemed to be buzzing. Funnily enough Graham and Kevin in their basques, stockings and suspenders "Rocky Horror" costumes did not look at all out of place!! In fact, it was unusual that for once, a group of "disabled" walking down the street en masse was not the centre of attention! It was in fact the man in the stockings, suspenders, high heels, wig and full on make-up that turned the attention away from us. Thank you Graham, you may be disabled by association but you have your uses!

The only downside to that weekend was when we attempted to enter a restaurant in Grand Central Birmingham Station. They took one look at the group

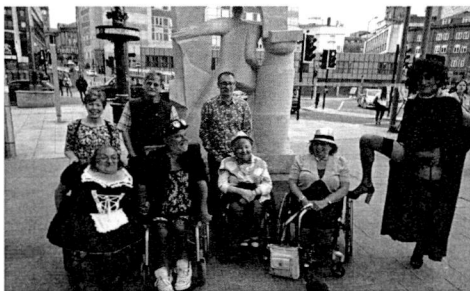

Trelorians hit Birmingham! Pride and Rocky Horror Show May 2019

and stated they couldn't accommodate us even though the place was only half full. I suspect they thought we would be slow eaters, and they wanted to close early!! From the restaurant next door we watched them close an hour and a half hour before the scheduled time as advertised on their website. We made a complaint to the companies Head Office, not just for being turned away but for the aggressive manner in which we were spoken to. We didn't like that fact we may have been discriminated against! The lady from Head Office handling our complaint was called Lina and she was most thorough in ensuring she had the facts straight. She viewed the CCTV and confirmed that we were indeed turned away two and a half hours before the restaurant was scheduled to close, and that the staff closed the restaurant an hour and a half early. The staff members were questioned by HR and the explanation they gave was that they had run out of prepped food. The CCTV showed they also turned away four other tables and we were told by Lina that this was completely against company policy. However, the CCTV did show that they then reopened again for the last hour – was this because as we left Graham shouted over "Just put you a review on Trip Adviser, thanks a lot" The company, by way of apology issued us with vouchers of £20 each. We retracted our theory that it was because we were disabled and realised it was just down to staff incompetence.

I began contemplating one day on why our little group "Get togethers" are so enjoyable. Graham doesn't socialise with any of his school friends from 40 plus years ago, and even if he did I doubt they would go away on weekend breaks together. I asked Liam and he said that he did keep contact with one old school friend but wouldn't dream of meeting up for a full weekend. I asked Kevin about his brother and he said pretty much the same thing. Yes contact, but probably not for overnight stays. The conclusion we have come to is this. We developed a very close bond all those years ago. We spent far more time with each other than my brother ever did with his friends. We were together 24/7 for months at a time. We came from all parts of the country and not just one village, town or even city. That bond is reflected by how, when we do meet up, we seem to know instinctively what each other's needs are. No one has to ask for help because, as at Treloars, we just got on with it and helped each other accepting one another's limitations. There is no embarrassment or awkwardness if I get stuck pushing myself up a hill, one of the others will just start shoving!

At the time of writing this book, the next trip has been sorted. I've sourced four purpose built lodges in Devon. Blagdon Farm boasts 100% purpose-built disabled accessible lakeside Lodges with fishing lakes accessed by easy wheelable paths and a swimming pool complete with hoist if required! We have also pre-booked Sunday dinner at the nearby Rydon Inn for that weekend. They didn't even flinch when Graham telephoned them and asked if they could accommodate six wheelchairs, seven walkers and five dogs!

Fingers crossed that it's all going to go to plan but if not I'm ready for the next challenge! My next book may be a travel guide specialising in breaks for those that appear on the outside to be "Disabled" but have forgotten to tell their brains that! It is after all, only accessibility that is the true "handicap", not the person.

Finally, my friend Janet and I once had a conversation where we discussed what we would change about ourselves if anything was possible. Janet said she would change her teeth as her medical condition causes her teeth to not be very strong.

I said I would like to be able to have feet that fitted into normal shoes.

Neither of us thought to say "To not have been born disabled"

Oh, and Graham is still my "Current husband"!

Acknowledgements

On 29th August 2018, my 57th birthday, exactly 57 years since that heat wave where the midwife indicated to my mum I may not survive, my son Christopher took me for breakfast in the Sky Garden at the "Walkie Talkie" building in London. He asked me what I was going to do with my life now that I'm no longer working. I said I'd always wanted to write about my life experiences. "So do it" he said. "There's nothing to stop you." And so I did. "Thank you "Chris Cross"

Thank you also to my husband Graham, firstly for keeping me supplied with copious amounts of G & T and wine (not at the same time) throughout the process of writing this book. Secondly for reading my drafts so many times that he never wants to hear the words "Crotch Height Perspective" again.

Thank you to all those that proof read and corrected my spelling and grammar and pointed out the fact that for the first couple of drafts none of it made any sense at all. Our Friends Kerry and Colin, Steve and Sheila, and my sister in law Sue - the other Mrs S Derham. Your feedback has been invaluable.

Thank you to my son Jonathon for your encouragement and support, hopefully you will have actually read it by now "Jon Jon"

Thank you to Lord Mayor Treloar and his daughter Florence, for their foresight many many years ago. Without you both I may never have the friends I have now and "Trelorians on Tour" would simply not exist.

Speaking of whom, thank you to "Team Trelorians" for helping me to make memories that I actually wanted to write about!! Roz, Ian, Kevin, Janet, Elizabeth, Liam, Beverley, Sally, Marie, Roland, Richard, Vanessa, Dean, Linda, Chris and Andy.

And to the late Mr Tom Stoyle, who never stopped trying to improve my quality of life with his numerous orthopaedic operations and positivity, thank you.

Lastly to my late parents, Bob and Jennifer Pollock, whose attitude towards disability, and the determination that I would lead a "normal" life, made me who I am today. Thank you xx

Crotch Height Perspective – It's just the way it is!

Special thanks to Jane Hurst, Teacher of Mathematics at Florence Treloar School from 1977 - for her permission to copy the below plans of the original Florence Treloar School in 1965. Jane's book "Treloar's One Hundred Years of Education" was invaluable in providing me with some of the facts and figures I have included in this book in the chapter "The Treloar years"

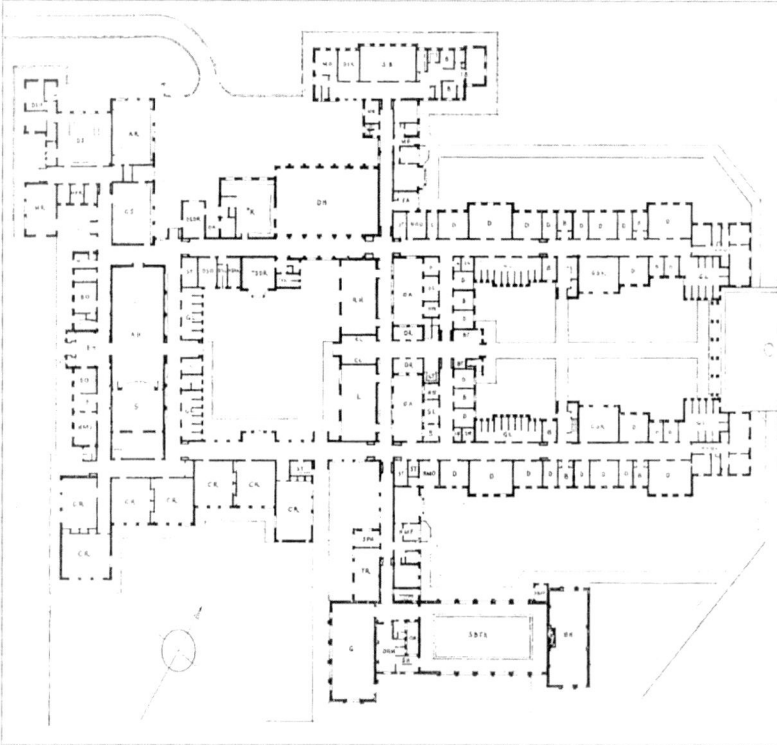

239

AH	Assembly Hall	HW	Hair Washing
AHMF	Assistant House Mistress' Flats	IB	Isolation Block
AR	Art Room	K	Kitchen
B	Bathroom	KSRR	Kitchen Staff Rest Room
BO	Bursar's Office	L	Library
BH	Boiler House	LN	Linen
BT	Boots	LT	Lift
C	Cleaners	MAO	Matron's Office
CL	Cloaks	MF	Matron's Flat
CR	Classrooms	ML	Men's Laboratory
D	Dormitories	MO	Medical Officer
DH	Dining Hall	MPR	Music Practice Room
DR	Drying Rooms	MR	Music Room
DS	Domestic Science	NN	Night Nurse
DSDR	Domestic Staff Dining Room	OA	Open Areas
DSIF	Domestic Science Instruction Flat	PG	Playground
DSL	Domestic Staff Lavatories	RR	Recreation Room
DSO	Domestic Superintendent's Office	S	Stage
DYR	Day Room	SB	Sick Bay
E	Enquiries	SBFP	Swimming Bath Filtration Plant
EH	Entrance Hall	SBTH	Swimming Bath
FA	First Aid	SH	Showers
G	Gymnasium	SL	Small Laundries
GL	Girls' Lavatories	SO	Secretary's Office
GS	General Science Laboratory	SPH	Speech Therapy
GSR	Girls' Sitting Rooms	ST	Stores
HMF	House Mistress' Flat	TR	Therapy
HMO	House Mistress' Office	TSDR	Teaching Staff Dining Room
HMS	Headmistress' Study	TSL	Teaching Staff Lavatories

240